Key Concepts in Public Policy

Student Workbook

Sally B. Solomon
Susan C. Roe

Key Concepts in Public Policy
Student Workbook

Sally B. Solomon, MSN, RN
Director, Public Policy and Research
National League for Nursing

Susan C. Roe, MS, RN
Consultant
Phoenix, Arizona

Pub. No. 15-1995A

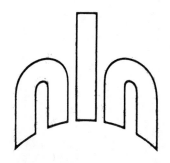

National League for Nursing • New York

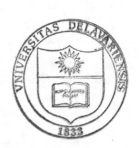

Preface

Key Concepts in Public Policy: Student Workbook is your key to basic knowledge and skills necessary to all nursing leaders. Knowledge of policy and politics and the power needed to implement sound policy are vital to nurses who are committed to meeting the health needs of the public. If nurses are to participate fully in decisions about the health care system of which they are so essential a part, they must understand the forces that influence that system, the actors who manipulate it, the ideas that shape it. The purpose of this book is to provide you with the information and skills you need to make an impact on the nation's health care.

Some parts of this book give you information—both factual knowledge and information about where to find out more about topics of interest. Other parts force you to be a participant. There are pen-and-pencil exercises you can use to make sure you have acquired basic content in policy and political structures, experiential exercises that introduce you to the policy-making process in a nonthreatening manner, and case studies and small-group exercises that allow you to apply all your skills. All the exercises draw on your nursing knowledge and experience to involve you in the policy process in ways that are most relevant to you.

This Workbook is designed to accompany a model course presented in *Integrating Public Policy into the Curriculum*, a handbook for instructors. It can be used either as an assigned text in an undergraduate curricular strand or master's level course, or as a self-study manual for nurses who are either in school or in a clinical setting. The Workbook consists of several sections that are intended to be used more or less simultaneously. The first section presents, in essay format, definitions and examples of key concepts in policy making and policy analysis. Next is an extensive Glossary of health care policy terms and government agencies. At the end of the book is a Resource List of books, newspapers and newsletters, journals, government publications, and other sources of interest to nurses studying public policy. Whether you are studying in class or alone, you will probably want to begin by familiarizing yourself with this information and the additional resources provided.

The middle sections of the Workbook consist of Exercises, Case Studies, and optional Small-Group Exercises, plus answers to the Exercises. The Exercises are divided into modules by main content areas, and subdivided into

Basic and Advanced Questions within each module. We hope that the Exercises will pique your interest by showing you the very many ways there are for nurses to make an impact on health care policy. The Case Studies and Small-Group Exercises give you additional opportunities to explore the complexities of policy making and the political process.

We wish to thank the following people for providing us with information: Michael Hash, Health Policy Alternatives, Inc.; Karen Ehrnman, American College of Nurse-Midwives; and Susan M. Jenkins, legal counsel to the District of Columbia Nurses' Association. They were of great help to us in making sure our factual details were correct; however, we are of course responsible for the accuracy of the final publication. We also thank Elaine Silverstein, our editor at NLN, for her patience, perseverance, and guidance throughout this project.

Sally B. Solomon
Susan C. Roe

Contents

Key Concepts in Public Policy

To effectively enter the world of policy and politics, it is essential that you understand some key concepts. These are defined in the following essay and are distinguished by **boldface** type.

A **policy** is a chosen course of action that has a significant effect on large numbers of people (MacRae & Wilde, 1979). In private organizations, policies may focus on such issues as hiring practices, personnel protocols (e.g., dress codes), or matters that pertain to the organization's product development and distribution or the delivery of its services. A policy is often developed in response to a problem, such as how a particular health care organization should respond to patients who require care but are unable to pay for services. The course of action chosen should be one that can be applied to equivalent situations over and over again (MacRae & Wilde, 1979).

In the public arena, policy decisions are typically responsive to societal problems (Nagel, 1984). Thus, a public policy is one that affects the safety and welfare of the population and determines how given amounts of resources will be utilized. For example, a health care policy that is now being acted out in the United States is the decision to make health care accessible (within certain parameters) to the elderly. The verbal commentary that describes this chosen course of action is called a **policy statement** (MacRae & Wilde, 1979). In this example, the chosen course of action has been translated into a **program** called Medicare.

The choice of action taken may ultimately require legislation or judicial or administrative decisions (MacRae & Wilde, 1979). For example, the policy problem of health and safety in the workplace resulted in the enactment of the Occupational Safety and Health Act (OSHA). Furthermore, programs or actions taken under the rubric of policy often have some type of approval mechanisms for entry or may carry some threat of sanction should the boundaries of the action not be adhered to. For example, in the Medicaid program (a health care financing program for the indigent), the criterion for participation is the use of an income test: the individual or family has to have less than a certain amount of money to be eligible for the program.

The goal of effective **policy making** is to address a variety of identified problems through a decision-making process that promotes the best decision by assessing the consequences of chosen courses of action. If the action is decided by society for itself or for society by its elected representatives, then a **public policy** is being considered (Quade, 1982). Public policy focuses on a range of problems affecting the population at large (Nagel, 1984). These problems may include needed actions in such areas as defense, business, the international marketplace, education, or foreign affairs. Therefore, health care is only one of the many societal problems that require attention by policy makers.

At the foundation of policy making is **policy analysis.** It is the process whereby logic, reason, and factual information are used to determine which public policy among a number of alternative policies will achieve desired goals (Nagel, 1984). Through policy analysis, one attempts to bring about better solutions to societal problems (Quade, 1982). The reasons for analyzing public policy is to determine what governments ought to do about identified problems: what action to take, how the government should implement that action for large segments of the population, or how the government should bring about changes in what is already being done. As a result, policy analysis can be either proactive or reactive (in other words, one may analyze prospective policies or policies that are already in place). Reactive analysis often takes the form of **program evaluation.**

Those who assess policy problems are called **policy analysts.** Policy analysts are usually people from the academic world or private sector, employees of the executive branch of government, or certain legislative staff members. Policy analysts attempt to provide **policy makers** (those who determine the action) with whatever information is needed and available so that, at the very least, the impact of both past and current public policies can be measured to determine whether policies should continue or new policies should be determined. Policy makers are legislators and government officials, plus executive branch people whose job it is to write regulations.

A policy analyst uses many approaches to assess policy problems (Brewer & deLeon, 1983). At times the approach used by a policy analyst may not meet the needs of the policy maker, who is often a legislator. The policy analyst may want to use a sophisticated technique or test the problem against theoretical assumptions, whereas the policy maker may be confronted with a pressing societal problem that needs quick analysis (Dye, 1976). Therefore, it has been found that for policy makers and analysts to be most effective, they must be aware of:

1. The desired goals of the new or existing policy or problem. For example, a desired goal may be that day care centers be provided for working women.

2. Possible ways of reaching the desired goal. For example, it may be possible to consider both public and private financing of day care centers.

3. Potential consequences for each policy alternative. For example, what will be the consequences of using either type of financing? What type of day care center is most appropriate?

4. Specific criteria that can be used to rank policy alternatives. For example, evaluate the effectiveness of day care centers by projecting the absenteeism rates of working mothers who are able to utilize the centers (Quade, 1982).

One helpful way of understanding policy analysis is to consider policy as an output (Lynn, 1980). In this sense, there are two possible approaches to consider—the incrementalist and rationalist models. From the standpoint of political feasibility, the **incrementalist approach** is the most expedient, since incrementalism does not require any major changes in financing and social values (Henry, 1980). Medicaid could be considered an incrementalist policy action, since only one population group was selected as the target for action and the methods used for financing the delivery of health care followed accepted practices. In the incrementalist model, new policies are only variations of old ones, and those policies are accepted as satisficing and legitimate. **Satisficing** refers to minimum goal achievement. Policies are designed to achieve only a narrowly defined goal. The decisions that are made only satisfy and suffice; they do not maximize. A drawback of the incrementalist model is that once substantial resources have been invested in existing programs, it tends to prevent the development of innovative new policies.

Under the **rationalist model,** one approaches policy analysis by looking at all possible preferences and alternatives, developing criteria for assessment, and in the process of decision making, calculating costs and benefits. In this model, one's goal is "better" policies (Henry, 1980). One method utilized in this model is **benefit-cost analysis,** the assessment and comparison of potential benefits or payoffs and known costs (Nagel, 1984). For example, in deciding whether to install air bags in automobiles as a means of reducing mortality in car accidents, the cost of the installation would be weighed against how many lives might be saved.

Because policy makers are concerned with feasibility and practicality, policy analysts would do well to keep these criteria in mind. The following guidelines should be used when analyzing policy:

1. Defining the scope of the problem. For instance, if the concern is health care, is the problem access to health care for the poor or health care for the nation? It is important to be aware of a tendency at this point of analysis to **suboptimize.** Suboptimizing is defining the problem too narrowly or considering only a part of the problem, which may result from intentful neglect or making incorrect assumptions.

2. Developing clear and consistent criteria by which the policies can be judged. **Effectiveness** (achievement of the desired goals or quantity of benefits) and **efficiency** (ratio of benefits to costs) are typical criteria of choice in policy analysis, along with **equity** (giving a benefit to many according to a criterion of fairness) and **ethics** (societal standards of right and wrong) (Nagel, 1984; MacRae & Wilde, 1979). For instance, under the notion of equity one might contend that all segments of the population should be provided with a minimum level of income, education, freedom from crime, or other goods that a government or society can allocate (Nagel, 1984). Therefore, one would ask whether **distributive justice**—spreading the benefit of the policy action so that no one group suffers—should be used as a criterion or whether ethical and philosophical premises (such as assessing the quality of human life) should be used. The problem at this stage is developing some standard of rightness. A policy dilemma now being faced that relates to criteria of choice is in determining who shall benefit from high technology. Should an enormous amount of resources be expended for one artificial heart recipient, or should these same resources be redistributed so that many are able to benefit?

3. Identifying a range of alternatives that will achieve desired policy goals, minimize any untoward effects on the particular group being affected, and circumvent political barriers. A variety of techniques may be employed to achieve these ends. It is at this point in the process of policy analysis that an incrementalist or rationalist approach may be taken.

4. Choosing a course of action that will have the best chance of being implemented in a political environment (feasibility). Society is comprised of a number of competing interest groups, and each group desires a particular course of action. It is the nature and scope of the conflict among these groups that sets the tone of the political environment.

Politics is the use of power or influence to obtain valued interests or desires. In policy analysis, determining the best policy choice may require intuitive judgment of the political environment rather than sophisticated technical analysis or factual information (MacRae & Wilde, 1979; Quade, 1982). For instance, oftentimes a potentially effective policy cannot be initiated because the political environment forbids it. Some would contend that the implementation of a national health insurance program has not been successful not only because of financing problems but also because of the tenor of the political environment.

Careful attention to the above steps can result in effective assessments of policy, whether it be the development of a new public policy or review and modification of an existing policy.

REFERENCES

Brewer, G.D., & deLeon, P. (1983). *The Foundations of Policy Analysis.* Homewood, IL: Dorsey Press.

Dye, T. R. (1976). *Policy Analysis: What Governments Do, Why They Do It, and What Difference It Makes.* University, AL: University of Alabama Press.

Henry, N. (1980). *Public Administration and Public Affairs.* Englewood Cliffs, NJ: Prentice-Hall.

Lynn, L. E., Jr. (1980). *Designing Public Policy.* Santa Monica, CA: Goodyear.

MacRae, D., Jr., & Wilde, J. A. (1979). *Policy Analysis for Public Decisions.* Boston, MA: Duxbury Press.

Nagel, S. S. (1984). *Public Policy: Goals, Means, and Methods.* New York: St. Martin's Press.

Quade, E. S. (1982). *Analysis for Public Decisions.* New York: Elsevier.

Glossary

Accreditation: the process by which an agency or organization evaluates and recognizes a program of study or an institution as meeting certain predetermined standards. Similar assessment of individuals is called **certification.** Accreditation is usually granted by a private organization created for the purpose of assuring the public of the quality of the accredited body, such as the NLN accreditation of nursing schools and home health agencies. Accreditation may either be permanent once obtained or limited to a specific period of time (like NLN accreditation). Unlike **licensure,** accreditation is not a condition of lawful practice but is intended as an indication of high-quality practice.

Actual charge: the amount a physician or other practitioner actually bills a patient for a particular medical service or procedure. The actual charge may differ from the **customary,** prevailing, or **reasonable charges** under Medicare and other insurance programs.

Aid to Families with Dependent Children (AFDC): a program jointly funded by the federal and state governments that provides cash assistance to very low income single-parent families with dependent children. Each state sets its own eligibility levels and chooses which federally defined groups it will cover. Most states limit coverage to single-parent families. AFDC recipients automatically receive Medicaid.

Allowable charge: the maximum fee that a third party will recognize in reimbursing a provider for a given service; in effect, the amount paid.

Allowable costs: items or elements of an institution's costs that are reimbursable under a cost-based payment formula. Before the implementation of Medicare's prospective payment system, hospitals were reimbursed on an allowable-cost basis. Medicare still reimburses skilled nursing facilities and home health agencies for their allowable costs.

Ancillary services: hospital or other inpatient services other than room and board and professional services. These may include X-ray examinations, drugs, and laboratory or other services separately itemized.

Appropriations bill: a measure enacted by Congress that sets the precise amount of funds to finance specific agencies or programs. This legislation permits federal agencies to incur obligations and to make payments from the Treasury for specified purposes. An appropriations bill usually follows authorizing legislation. The House, under the Constitution, initiates all appropriations bills, which must be signed into law by the President.

Area Health Education Center (AHEC): an organization or system of health, educational, and service institutions whose policy and programs are frequently under the direction of a medical school or university health science center and whose prime goals are to improve the distribution, supply, quality, utilization, and efficiency of health personnel in relation to specific medically underserved areas. AHECs receive federal funding for some of their operations.

Assignment: an agreement in which a patient assigns to another party, usually a provider, the right to receive payment from a third party for the service the patient has received. Assignment is used instead of a patient paying directly for the service and then receiving reimbursement from public or private insurance programs. Under Medicare, if a physician accepts assignment from the patient, he must agree to accept the program payment as payment in full (except for specific coinsurance, copayment, and deductible amounts required of the patient).

Authorization bill: a legislative prerequisite for an appropriations bill. An authorization bill is legislation enacted by Congress to initiate or continue a federal agency or program. It signifies approval of a program, establishes program policies, and puts a ceiling on monies that can be used to finance it. Once an authorization bill is passed, the appropriations process results in the determination of the actual amount of funds that will be available.

Beneficiary: a person who is eligible to receive, or who is receiving, benefits from an insurance policy or government entitlement program, such as Medicare.

Blue Cross/Blue Shield plans: nonprofit health plans guaranteeing payment for covered care and offered by autonomous corporations originally founded by hospitals and physicians. They sell health insurance similar to that offered by commercial insurance companies. Blue Cross covers hospitalization and Blue Shield covers physician services.

Budget process: the annual federal process by which aggregate fiscal resources are allocated among government agencies and programs in the budget.

Budget resolution: Two resolutions initiated and passed by Congress are used for the federal budget. The first budget resolution establishes an interim guideline for the budget and is to be reported to and adopted by the House and Senate by June 15. The second budget resolution reaffirms or revises the first resolution, is due September 15, and is legally binding.

Capital: plant or equipment used in the production of goods and services, the value of such assets, or money specifically available for their acquisition or development. This includes, for example, the buildings, beds, and equipment used in the provision of hospital services.

Capital depreciation: the decline in value of capital assets (assets of a permanent or fixed nature, goods and plant) over time with use.

Capitation: a method of payment for health services in which an individual or institutional provider is paid a fixed amount for each person served without regard to the actual number or nature of services provided to each person. Capitation is characteristic of health maintenance organizations and other alternative delivery systems.

Carrier: a commercial health insurer, a government agency, or a Blue Cross or Blue Shield plan that underwrites or administers programs that pay for health services. Under Medicare Part B (Supplemental Medical Insurance) and the Federal Employees Health Benefits Program, carriers are agencies and organizations with which the program contracts for administration of various functions, including payment of claims.

Case management: a system under which the recipient of health services must have all services approved by a case manager (can be a physician, clinic, or nurse, who is usually also the primary provider of care).

Case mix: the diagnosis-specific makeup of a health care provider's patient population. Case mix is reflected in patients' lengths of stay as well as the intensity, cost, and scope of the services provided by a hospital or other health program.

Catchment area: a geographic area defined and served by a health program or institution such as a hospital or community mental health center delineated on the basis of such factors as population density, natural geographic boundaries, political boundaries, accessibility of transportation, and economic patterns.

Categorically needy: persons who are eligible to receive public assistance. Under Medicaid, such categories include the aged, blind, disabled, and families with children under 18 (or 21, if in school) in which one parent is absent, disabled, or unemployed; in addition, the categories include specific income and asset requirements.

Center for Disease Control (CDC): organization within the Department of Health and Human Services (DHHS) serving as a focal point for disease control and public health activities. The Center provides facilities and services for the investigation, prevention, and control of diseases.

Certificate of need (CON): a certificate issued by a government body to an individual or organization proposing to build or modify a health facility or offer a new or different service. This certificate recognizes that such facility of service will be needed by those for whom it is intended, and is meant to prevent excessive or duplicative development of facilities and services. The **health systems agencies** are required to make recommendations to the state agencies regarding proposed new institutional health services within their areas.

Certification: the process by which a nongovernmental agency or association grants recognition to an individual who has met certain predetermined qualifications specified by that agency or association.

Civilian Health and Medical Program of the Uniformed Services (CHAMPUS): a program, administered by the Department of Defense, without premiums but with cost-sharing provisions, that pays for care delivered to retired members and dependents of active and retired members of the seven uniformed services of the United States (Army, Navy, Air Force, Marine Corps, Commissioned Corps of the Public Health Service, Coast Guard, and the National Oceanic and Atmospheric Administration).

Claims-incurred policy: the conventional form of malpractice insurance, under which the insured is covered for any claims arising from an incident that occurred or is alleged to have occurred during the policy period, regardless of when the claim is made. The only limiting factors are the statutes of limitations, which vary from state to state. An alternative type of policy is the **claims-made policy.**

Claims-made policy: a form of malpractice insurance gaining increasing popularity among insurers because it increases the accuracy of ratemaking. Under this type of policy, the insured is covered for any claim made, rather than any injury occurring, while the policy is in force. Claims made after the insurance lapses are not covered, as they are by a **claims-incurred policy.** Claims-made policies were initially resisted by providers because of the nature of medical malpractice claims, which may arise several years after an injury occurs. A retired physician, for example, could be sued but not be covered, unless special provisions are made to continue his coverage beyond his years of practice.

Coinsurance: a cost-sharing requirement under public or private health insurance that provides that the insured will assume a fixed percentage of the cost of covered services.

Conference committee: a committee comprised of members of both houses of Congress that resolves differences on pieces of legislation or policy. Members of conference committees are drawn from the senior members of the committees that originally considered the legislation. Conference committees consider bills that have been approved by both houses, and their recommendations must be adopted by each house before action by the President.

Congressional Budget Office (CBO): a nonpartisan agency that provides Congress with budget-related information and analyses, including comments on alternative fiscal policies.

Consumer price index (CPI): an economic index prepared by the Bureau of Labor Statistics of the U.S. Department of Labor. It measures the change in average prices of the goods and services purchased by urban wage earners and clerical workers and their families. It is widely used as an indicator of changes in the cost of living, as a measure of inflation (and deflation, if any) in the economy, and as a means for studying trends in prices of various goods and services. The CPI is made up of several components, which measure prices in different sectors of the economy. One of these, the medical care component, gives trends in medical care charges based on specific indicators of hospital, medical, dental, and drug prices.

Continuing resolution: in the federal

budget, legislation enacted by Congress to provide spending authority for specific ongoing activities in a fiscal year in cases where the regular appropriation for such activities has not been enacted by the beginning of the fiscal year.

Copayment: a type of cost sharing whereby insured or covered persons pay a specified flat amount per unit of service or unit of time (e.g., $2 per visit, $10 per inpatient hospital day), and their insurer payes the rest of the cost. The copayment is incurred at the time the service is used.

Cost-related or cost-based reimbursement: one method of payment to medical care programs by third parties, typically Blue Cross plans (formerly Medicare), for services delivered to patients. In cost-related systems, the amount of the payment is based on the costs to the provider of delivering the service.

Credentialing: a generic term referring to **accreditation, certification,** and **licensure** and the formal recognition of professional or technical competence.

Customary charge: generally, the amount a physician normally or usually charges the majority of his patients. Under Medicare, it is the median charge by a particular physician for a specific type of service. Customary charges, in addition to actual and prevailing charges, are taken into account in determining reasonable charges for physicians under Medicare.

Deductible: the amount of loss or expense that must be incurred by an insured individual before an insurer will assume any liability for the remaining cost of covered services. Deductibles may be either fixed dollar amounts or the value of specified services (such as two days of hospital care or one physician visit).

Diagnosis Related Groups (DRGs): 471 categories of illness into which patients with similar clinical conditions are placed, and for which average payment rates are preestablished. Medicare and some other insurers now pay for hospital services according to DRG classification.

Division of Nursing: the major office of nursing affairs within the federal government. The Division of Nursing is a unit of the Bureau of Health Professions Education of the Health Resources Services Administration, located within the Public Health Service of the DHHS. The Division focuses on and supports nursing education, practice, and some research under the authority of the Nurse Education Act.

Early and Periodic Screenings, Diagnosis, and Treatment Program (EPSDT): a required component of the Medicaid program in which states must provide or arrange medical services for eligible children under the age of 21. Services are to include identification of physical and mental health problems and all treatment necessary to cure or ameliorate those problems. The states have an outreach obligation that includes educating eligible persons about the available benefits and assisting them in obtaining needed care.

Federal fiscal year: the twelve-month period from October 1 to September 30.

Fee-for-service: method of charging whereby a physician or other practitioner bills for each encounter or service rendered.

Department of Health and Human Services (DHHS): the department within the executive branch of government responsible for administering the government's health and human services programs. Headed by the Secretary of DHHS, the major agencies within the department include the Public Health Service, the Health Care Financing Administration, the Social Security Administration, and the Office of Human Development Services. It also includes the Food and Drug Administration and the Center for Disease Control.

First-dollar coverage: coverage under an insurance policy that begins with the first dollar of expense incurred by the insured for the covered benefits. Such coverage, therefore, has no **deductible,** although it may have **copayments** or **coinsurance.**

Fiscal intermediary or **fiscal agent:** a contractor that processes and pays provider claims on behalf of Medicare or a state Medicaid agency.

Fiscal year: any twelve-month period for which annual accounts are kept. Sometimes, but by no means necessarily, the same as a calendar year. See **federal fiscal year.**

General Accounting Office (GAO): a staff agency of Congress that serves as the investigating agency for Congress in legal, accounting, and other fiscal areas. Its recommendations are intended to make for more effective government operations, and to ensure the proper expenditure, control, and accountability for government funds.

Grandfather clause or provision: a clause or provision of law that permits continued eligibility or coverage for individuals or organizations receiving program benefits under the law despite a change in the law that would otherwise make them ineligible or that in some other manner exempts a person, organization, or thing from a change in law that would otherwise effect him or it.

Health Care Financing Administration (HCFA): the agency within the Department of Health and Human Services that is responsible for administering the Medicare and Medicaid programs. Activities include issuing regulations, providing matching funds to states for administering Medicaid, compiling data, establishing standards, contracting with peer review organizations and fiscal intermediaries and carriers, and monitoring quality and cost.

Health maintenance organization (HMO): an entity with four essential attributes: (1) an organized system for providing health care in a geographic area that provides or otherwise ensures the delivery of (2) an agreed-upon set of basic and supplemental health maintenance and treatment services to (3) a voluntarily enrolled group of persons (4) for which the HMO is reimbursed through predetermined, fixed, periodic prepayment made by or on behalf of each person or family unit enrolled in the HMO without regard to the amount of actual services provided.

Health manpower: collectively, all men and women working in the provision of health services, whether as individual practitioners or employees of health institutions and programs; whether or not professionally trained; and whether or not subject to public regulation. Facilities and manpower are the principal health resources used in producing health services.

Health Resources and Services Administration (HRSA): located within the Public Health Service, HRSA administers federal programs related to direct health delivery, target populations, and health planning. It also supports and conducts research on health personnel, including nurses.

Health systems agency (HSA): a health planning and resource development agency that exists in many health services areas in the United States. HSA functions, legislated by the National Health Planning and Resources Development Act of 1974, include preparation of a health services plan (HSP) and an annual implementation plan (AIP), issuance of grants and contracts, the initial review and approval or disapproval of proposed uses of a wide range of federal funds in the agency's health service area, and review of proposed new and existing institutional health services.

Hill-Burton Act: a program pursuant to federal legislation whereby hospitals and other medical facilities received federal grants and loans for building or modernization, and in return incurred certain obligations. The uncompensated care obligation required facilities that received Hill-Burton funds to provide a certain amount of free or reduced-cost care to persons unable to pay, for a period of twenty years. The community service obligation, which continues forever, requires Hill-Burton facilities to provide emergency care to all persons without regard to ability to pay and to provide all of the facility's services to the general public (including Medicare and Medicaid patients) without discrimination.

Home health agency: an agency that provides home health care. To be certified under Medicare, an agency must provide skilled nursing services and at least one additional therapeutic service (physical, speech, or occupational therapy, medical social services, or home health aide services) in the home.

Home health care: health services rendered to an individual as needed in the home. Such services are provided to aged, disabled, or sick or convalescent individuals who do not need institutional care. The services may be provided by a visiting nurse association (VNA), home health agency, hospital, or other organized community group. They may be quite specialized or comprehensive (nursing services; speech, physical, occupational, and rehabilitation therapy; homemaker services; and social services).

Homemaker services: nonmedical support services (e.g., food preparation, bathing) given a homebound individual who is unable to perform these tasks himself. Such services are not covered under the Medicare and Medicaid program (unless the patient meets

...itions for home care eligibility) ...ealth insurance programs, but ...¹ in the social service programs ...e states under Title XX of the ...ct. Homemaker services are ...ve independent living and ...y life for aged, disabled, sick, or ...valescent people.

Hospice: a program that provides palliative and supportive care for terminally ill patients and their families, either directly or on a consulting basis with the patient's physician or another community agency such as a visiting nurse association.

Independent practice association (IPA): a type of HMO in which the physicians are organized independent of the HMO and contract with the HMO to provide their services, often on a **fee-for-service** basis, from their own offices while continuing their private practice.

Indirect cost: a cost that cannot be identified directly with a particular activity, service, or product of the program experiencing the cost. Indirect costs are usually apportioned among the program's services in proportion to each service's share of direct costs.

Infant mortality: the death (mortality) of live-born children who have not reached their first birthday, usually measured as a rate: number of infant deaths per 1,000 live births in a given area or program during a given time period. The infant mortality rate is one common measure of health status of a community.

Institute of Medicine (IOM): the IOM was chartered in 1970 by the National Academy of Sciences to enlist distinguished members of the medical and other professions for the examination of policy matters pertaining to the health of the public. In this, the Institute acts under both the Academy's 1863 Congressional charter as an advisor to the federal government and on its own initiative in identifying issues of medical care, research, and education.

Institutional licensure: a proposed licensure system under which medical care institutions would be generally licensed by the state and would then be free to hire and use personnel as each saw fit, whether or not they met usual requirements for individual licensure. Under this system, formal education would become only one of many criteria used in assigning employees to particular positions.

Intermediary: see **fiscal intermediary.**

Intermediate care facility (ICF): an institution recognized under the Medicaid program and licensed under state law to provide, on a regular basis, health-related care and services to individuals who do not require the degree of care or treatment a hospital or skilled nursing facility is designed to provide but who, because of their mental or physical condition, require care and services above the level of room and board that can be made available to them only through institutional facilities. Public institutions for care of the mentally retarded or people with related conditions are also included.

Joint Commission on Accreditation of Hospitals (JCAH): a private, nonprofit organization whose purpose is to encourage the attainment of uniformly high standards of institutional medical care.

Licensure: the process by which an agency of government grants permission to an individual to engage in a given occupation upon finding that the applicant has attained the degree of competence necessary to ensure that the public health, safety, and welfare will be reasonably well protected.

Lobbying: efforts, including the provision of information, argument, or other means, by anybody other than a citizen acting on his own behalf to influence a governmental official in the performance of his duty.

Malpractice: professional misconduct or lack of ordinary skill in the performance of a professional act. A practitioner is liable for damages or injuries caused by malpractice. Such liability, for some professions, can be covered by malpractice insurance against the costs of defending suits instituted against the professional or any damages assessed by the court, usually up to a maximum limit. Malpractice requires that the patient demonstrate some injury and that the injury be caused by negligence.

Mark-up: the process of writing the actual language of a bill, done in committee after hearings are held. At this point in the legislative process, a bill may be altered, amended, rewritten, or entirely blocked (killed).

Medicaid (Title XIX): a medical assistance program started in 1965 and funded jointly by the federal government and the states. Medicaid reimburses providers for some institutional and ambulatory care services, which differ widely in amount from state to state. Medicaid is available to most recipients of **AFDC** and **SSI** and, in some states, to very low income persons with high medical bills.

Medically indigent: a person who is too impoverished to meet his medical expenses. It may refer either to persons whose income is low enough that they can pay for their basic living costs but not their routine medical care or to persons with generally adequate incomes who suddenly face catastrophically large medical bills.

Medicare (Title XVIII): a nationwide health insurance program for people aged 65 and over, for persons eligible for Social Security disability payments for over two years, and for others who suffer from end-stage renal disease. Health insurance protection is available to insured persons without regard to income. Monies from payroll taxes and premiums from beneficiaries are deposited in special trust funds for use in meeting the expenses incurred by the insured. The program was enacted on July 30, 1965, as Title XVIII—Health Insurance for the Aged—of the Social Security Act, and became effective on July 1, 1966. It consists of two separate but coordinated programs: hospital insurance (Part A), and supplementary medical insurance (Part B). Part A is funded mainly by a small payroll tax on employers and employees, whereas Part B is funded with premiums paid by Medicare recipients and federal revenues. Medicare recipients have substantial cost-sharing obligations in the form of deductibles and coinsurance under both Parts A and B.

Medigap policy: a health insurance policy designed to supplement limitations of Medicare coverage.

Morbidity: the extent of illness, injury, or disability in a defined population. It is usually expressed in general or specific rates of incidence or prevalence. Sometimes used to refer to any episode of disease.

Mortality: death. The mortality rate (death rate) expresses the number of deaths in a unit of population within a prescribed time.

National Center for Nursing Research: enacted in 1985 as part of the NIH reauthorization bill, this agency is to include research activities formerly conducted by the Division of Nursing in HRSA and is to be the focal point for all nursing research within the federal government. Its purpose is to better integrate nursing research with other biomedical and health care research at NIH and across the country.

National Health Service Corps: a program administered by the U.S. Public Health Service that provides assistance for individuals preparing for the health professions and obligates them to serve in areas with a critical shortage of health care workers for the purpose of improving the delivery of health care and services to persons residing in those areas.

National Institutes of Health (NIH): located within the Public Health Service and situated in Bethesda, Maryland, NIH supports and conducts over $4 billion annually of intramural and extramural biomedical research related to the causes and prevention of diseases. The Library of Medicine and the National Center for Nursing Research are part of NIH.

Nonprofit hospital: a general acute-care hospital whose earnings do not inure to the benefit of any private shareholder or individual. (Profits are used for capital expansion, new equipment, etc.)

Office of Management and Budget (OMB): responsible for managing and administering the budget for the departments within the executive branch of government. OMB consolidates and makes the final decisions on each department's annual budget requests and prepares the President's annual budget proposal. OMB also reviews all federal government regulations and coordinates all of the Administration's legislative initiatives and policy statements.

Office of Technology Assessment (OTA): a staff agency of Congress that provides information and analyses to Congress on the political, physical, economic, and social effects of technological applications, including health care technology.

Pocket veto: occurs when a bill is sent to the President while Congress is in adjournment *without* any fixed date for reconvening. If the President fails to sign the bill within ten days, the bill is pocket vetoed, and the veto cannot be overridden.

Preferred provider organization (PPO): an arrangement between health care providers, private or government insurers, and insured persons in which fees are reduced for insured persons using the PPO providers. PPOs usually provide reduced premiums because of their reliance on a network of lower-cost providers.

Premium: the amount of money paid by an insured person (or on his behalf) to an insurer or third party for insurance coverage.

Primary care: basic or general health care which emphasizes the point at which the patient first seeks assistance from the health care system and the care for the simpler and more common illnesses. The primary care provider usually also assumes ongoing responsibility for the patient in both health maintenance and therapy of illness. Primary care, as understood by nurses, is comprehensive in the sense that it takes responsibility for the overall coordination of care of the patient's health problems, be they biological, behavioral, or social.

Professional liability: obligation of providers or their professional liability insurers to pay for damages resulting from the providers' acts of omission or commission in treating patients. The term is sometimes preferred by providers to medical malpractice because it does not necessarily imply negligence. It is also a term that more adequately describes the obligations of all types of professions, such as lawyers, architects, and other health providers, as well as physicians and nurses.

Proprietary (for-profit) hospital: a hospital operated for the purpose of making a profit for its owners. Proprietary hospitals are often owned by physicians for the care of their own and others' patients. There is also a growing number of investor-owned hospitals, usually operated by parent corporations that operate chains of such hospitals.

Prospective Payment Assessment Commission (ProPAC): a congressionally mandated commission directed to make recommendations to Congress regarding Medicare's prospective payment system (PPS). Some of the areas it is responsible for include recalibration of DRG weights, the impact of technology on PPS, the impact of PPS on the quality of care, annual changes in the DRG rates, and other ongoing needs for revision of the PPS.

Prospective payment system (PPS): Medicare's new system of payment for inpatient hospital care in which hospitals are paid prospectively determined rates according to DRG on a per discharge basis. The PPS is intended to contain costs by creating an incentive for hospitals to operate more efficiently: if the hospital's cost is less than the prospective payment rate, it keeps the difference, while it receives no additional reimbursement if its costs exceed the payment rate.

Prospective reimbursement: any method of paying hospitals or other health programs in which amounts or rates of payment are established in advance of the provision of service and the providers are paid these amounts regardless of the costs they actually incur. These systems of reimbursement are designed to put providers of service at financial risk for the volume of services they provide.

Provider: an individual or institution that gives medical care. Under Medicare, institutional providers include hospitals, skilled nursing facilities, home health agencies, and certain providers of outpatient physical therapy services.

Public Health Service (PHS): part of the Department of Health and Human Services that establishes national health policy regarding the protection and advancement of physical and mental health. Its many agencies work together to administer programs that develop health resources and improve the delivery of health services. They also work to prevent communicable diseases and to conduct and support health care research.

Public hospital: a hospital owned and operated by a city, county, state, or federal government.

Reasonable charge: the amount, subject to a deductible and coinsurance, that Medicare will pay for a physician's service.

Recission: in the federal budget, enacted legislation cancelling budget authority previously provided by Congress. Recissions proposed by the President must be transmitted in a special message to Congress.

Reinsurance: the practice of one insurance company buying insurance from a second company for the purpose of protecting itself against part or all of the losses it might incur in the process of honoring the claims of its policyholders. The original company is called the ceding company; the second is the assuming company or reinsurer. Reinsurance may be sought by the ceding company for several reasons: to protect itself against losses in individual cases beyond a certain amount, where competition requires it to offer policies providing coverage in excess of these amounts; to offer protection against catastrophic losses in a certain line of insurance, such as aviation accident insurance; or to protect against mistakes in rating and underwriting in entering a new line of insurance, such as major medical.

Reliability: in research, the reproducibility of an experimental result; i.e., how closely a second study would yield the same results, whether or not they are correct.

Retrospective reimbursement: payment to providers by a third-party carrier for costs or charges actually incurred by subscribers in a previous time period. This method of hospital payment was traditionally used by Medicare.

Rural health clinic: a primary-care clinic located in a rural area, defined by the Rural Health Clinic Services Act, which authorized reimbursement of services under Medicaid and Medicare on a reasonable cost-related basis. The Act also authorized reimbursement for nurse practitioners and physician assistants working with the supervision, but not necessarily the on-site presence, of a physician.

Self-insurance: The practice of an individual, group of individuals, employer, or organization assuming complete responsibility for losses that might be insured against, such as malpractice losses, or medical expenses and other losses due to illness. Self-insurance is contrasted to the practice of purchasing insurance, by the payment of a premium, from some third party (an insurance company or government agency).

Skilled nursing facility (SNF): under Medicare and Medicaid, an institution (or a distinct part of an institution) that has in effect a transfer agreement with one or more participating hospitals and that (1) is primarily engaged in providing skilled nursing care and related services for patients who require medical or nursing care, or rehabilitation services for the rehabilitation of injured, disabled, or sick persons; (2) has formal policies, developed with the advice of a group of professional personnel, including one or more physicians and one or more registered nurses, to govern the skilled nursing care and related

medical or other services it provides; (3) has a physician, a registered professional nurse, or a medical staff responsible for the execution of such policies; (4) has a requirement that the health care of every patient be under the supervision of a physician, and provides for having a physician available to furnish necessary medical care in case of an emergency; (5) maintains medical records on all patients; and (6) provides 24-hour nursing service and has at least one registered professional nurse employed full-time.

Supplemental Security Income (SSI): a federal program, established under Title XVI of the Social Security Act, that provides cash assistance to low-income persons who are aged, blind, or disabled. In most states, SSI recipients generally receive Medicaid. In about fifteen states, they must meet more restrictive standards.

Supplementary Medical Insurance Program (Medicare Part B, SMI): the voluntary portion of Medicare in which all persons entitled to the hospital insurance program (Part A) may enroll. The program is financed on a current basis from monthly premiums paid by person insured under the program and the remaining amount from federal general revenues.

Teaching hospital: a hospital that provides undergraduate or graduate medical education, usually with one or more medical, dental, or osteopathic internship and residency programs and affiliation with a medical school. Hospitals that educate nurses and other health personnel but do not train physicians are not generally thought of as teaching hospitals, nor are those that have only programs of continuing education for practicing professionals.

Third-party payer: any organization, public or private, that pays or insures health or medical expenses on behalf of beneficiaries or recipients (e.g., Blue Cross and Blue Shield, commercial insurance companies, Medicare, and Medicaid). In all private and some public programs, the individual pays a premium for such coverage.

Title XVIII: see **Medicare.**

Title XIX: see **Medicaid.**

Trust funds: funds collected and used by the federal government for carrying out specific purposes and programs according to the terms of a trust agreement or statute, such as the social security and unemployment trust funds.

Usual, customary, and reasonable plans (UCR): health insurance plans that pay a provider's full charge if (1) it does not exceed his or her usual charge; (2) it does not exceed the amount customarily charged for the service by most other physicians in the area; or (3) it is otherwise reasonable.

Utilization review (UR): evaluation of the necessity, appropriateness, and quality of medical services, procedures, and facilities. In a hospital, this includes review of the appropriateness of admissions, services ordered and provided, length of stay, and discharge practices, both on a concurrent and retrospective basis. Utilization review can be done by a utilization review committee, PRO, other peer review group, or public agency.

Validity: the degree to which data or results of a study are correct or true; the extent to which a situation as observed reflects the true situation.

Veto: bills that pass both houses of Congress require presidential approval before becoming law. The President has 10 working days (excluding Sundays) to sign or veto a bill. If the President vetos the bill, a two-thirds majority of each house of Congress is needed to override the bill. If the President fails to sign a bill while Congress is in session or while Congress is in adjournment with a fixed date for reconvening, the bill automatically becomes law. See also **pocket veto.**

Voluntary agency: any nonprofit, nongovernmental agency, governed by lay or professional individuals, organized on a national, state, or local basis, whose primary purpose is health-related.

Women, Infant, and Children Program (WIC): the Special Supplemental Food Program for Women, Infants, and Children, sponsored by the U.S. Department of Agriculture and designed to provide extra nutritious food for mothers, infants, and young children. Authorized by the Child Nutrition Act of 1966, the WIC program serves the nutritional needs of pregnant women, breastfeeding women, and children up to five years of age. The program is supported with funds from the federal government but is administered by state health departments and local WIC agencies.

Exercises

The following exercises are intended not as a test but as a learning experience. They are grouped into seven content areas, following the seven modules of the model public policy course laid out in the accompanying teacher's book, *Integrating Public Policy into the Curriculum.* Within each module, the questions are subdivided into basic and advanced exercises. The Basic Exercises test core content information that all nurses should have; baccalaureate students and practicing nurses without graduate degrees should be able to complete them with the help of reference books and the Glossary in this Workbook. Master's level students should also complete the Basic Exercises as a demonstration of basic competency in the areas of policy and politics before going on to the Advanced Exercises in each module.

Suggested answers to all exercises are provided in the next section of this book. In most cases, these are intended merely as guidelines; feel free to exercise your creativity and fashion innovative solutions to these problems. The exercises are intended to be challenging and to draw upon all of your nursing knowledge and skill, but also to allow you to begin to work on policy problems in a nonthreatening atmosphere. Many of the Advanced Exercises can be worked on by groups or pairs of students.

Refer to the Resource List at the end of this Workbook for books, journals, and other materials that will be helpful in answering these exercises.

I. Historical Evolution of Delivery of Health Care and Nursing

A. Basic Questions
   1. Give an example of how Florence Nightingale exemplified the potential of nurses as influencers of health care policy.

2. List three causes for the federal government's high health care bills.

3. Explain the current major justification for the federal government's expenditures on nursing education and research.

B. Advanced Questions

1. For each of the past three decades (1960s, 1970s, 1980s), describe the major focus of federal health care legislation.

2. Select an early political thinker (e.g., Hobbes, Rousseau, Locke, de Toqueville). Discuss his major ideas and how they influenced the development of American government.

3. Select a situation you have encountered in practice and show how it was caused or affected by a health policy issue and how knowledge of policy could help you to rectify the situation. For example, you might discuss one of the following situations:

    a. Helping a child gain access to preventive care requires knowledge of a state's EPSDT as well as other child health programs.

b. A problem with utilization review and pressure for early discharge might be alleviated by knowing how to work with a PRO.

II. Health Policy Analysis and Program Evaluation

A. Basic Questions

1. List three areas involving health policy analysis to which nurses are especially well-prepared to contribute because of their experience as health care providers (for example, quality of patient care, long-term care).

2. Outline the process of how a bill becomes a law on the federal level. Explain how nurses can intervene at specific points in the process.

3. What is the *Federal Register* and how does one obtain a copy? What does one need to know in order to comment on a set of federal regulations?

4. Discuss the roles of committees, committee staff members, and special-interest groups in health policy formulation.

B. Advanced Questions

1. Select a publicly financed program that involves health care delivery (e.g., End Stage Renal Disease, Medicaid, health maintenance organization program). Give three criteria to be used in evaluating the program so that results would be helpful in policy analysis.

2. Select two health delivery problems that you have encountered in your practice. Discuss how you would set priorities for resolving these problems in terms of government funding, assuming that there are limited funds and a choice must be made between the two. What factors must be considered in comparing the two programs and making the fairest and most reasonable choice in allocating limited resources? What models or theories can be used in your analysis? What factors should be considered in carrying out cost/benefit analysis for both approaches?
   Examples of problems you might choose are (choose either **a** or **b**):

   a. How to select the most effective means of prenatal care to reduce the need for costly neonatal intensive care facilities.

   b. Diabetes screening versus hypertension screening.

3. Discuss some of the most common problems in program evaluation and why often the findings of program evaluation are not effectively applied to policy implementation. For example, despite research documenting the success of nurse-midwives in lowering infant morbidity, they are still not considered as viable an alternative to obstetricians as one would expect.

III. *Politics and Economics of Health Care Financing*

A. Basic Questions

1. Select two government agencies that deal with health care financing and describe their function and placement within the federal government.

2. What is the difference between Medicare's current prospective payment and previous reasonable-cost reimbursement system?

3. What is the difference between authorizations and appropriations in the legislative process?

4. Pick one of the DRGs listed below. Give an example of how two patients within that DRG might require different nursing resources.

  a. 14—Specific cerebrovascular disorders except transient ischemic attacks.

  b. 121—Circulatory disorders with acute myocardial infarction and cerebrovascular complications, discharged alive.

  c. 294—Diabetes, age greater than or equal to 36.

  d. 355—Nonradical hysterectomy, age less than 70, without complications and comorbidities.

5. a. What is the difference between Medicare and Medicaid?

b. What is the difference between Medicare Part A and Part B?

c. What is the Tax Equity and Fiscal Responsibility Act (TEFRA), and how does it relate to DRGs?

B. Advanced Questions

1. Outline the federal budget process, making sure to include the role and function of the following:

Office of Management and Budget (OMB)
President
Congressional budget committees
House of Representatives and Senate
Congressional Budget Office (CBO)

2. Describe the difference between regulation and competition in health care economics. Discuss ways that both can be ascribed to Medicare's prospective payment system. Is the health care system more regulatory or competitive as a result of DRGs? Explain your answer.

3. Interview a nurse administrator in either an acute-care setting or community agency. What have been her greatest challenges under DRGs? How does she think things are better or worse for nurses? for patients? for the agency? What does she think will be the next policy developments for the Medicare population? Finally, pose two questions of your own relating to DRGs and health policy. Prepare a report of the interview.

4. You are to give half-hour talks to three different groups: nurses, elderly consumers, and legislators. For each audience, what are the five most important points you will make on the politics and economics of health care financing?

IV. Alternative Delivery Systems: Issues and Problems

A. Basic Questions

1. Define: primary care, health maintenance organization, independent practice association, preferred provider organization.

2. Discuss the advantages and disadvantages of health maintenance organizations, preferred provider organizations, urgent care centers, and birthing centers from the consumer's point of view.

3. What is the status of direct third-party reimbursement for nurses in your state? Is it different for nurses with different types of specialization (e.g., nurse practitioners, nurse-midwives, psych/mental health nurses)?

B. Advanced Questions

1. What is the difference between vertical and horizontal integration? Give an example of each.

2. Select a current legislative proposal or recently enacted law that promotes an alternative health care delivery system. Describe the content and major purpose of the bill. Who were the original sponsors? At what point is it in the legislative process? What are the pros and cons of the bill? its chances of enactment? implications for nursing?
At the time of writing, examples one might choose are:
    Community Nursing Centers Bill
    Medicare's voucher system

3. Select a patient you have encountered whose situation demonstrates the fragmentation of services within the health care system, especially for Medicare patients. Explain what could be done to alleviate the problem.

4. Contact a major third-party payer (Blue Cross-Blue Shield or an insurance company) and a major employer in your community. What is each doing in the area of prevention? What areas of coverage do they provide in their policies that they did not provide in the past?

What areas of coverage have been cut back? What data do they collect? What coalitions are they part of? What are their impressions of nurses and third-party reimbursement for nurses? Prepare a report on the information you obtain.

V. *Technological, Legal, and Ethical Dimensions of Health Policy*

A. Basic Questions

1. List three government agencies involved with new technology in the field of health care. State the function of each agency and which branch of government it is part of.

2. What are two areas of state legislation that pertain to nursing practice? What are the specific laws on these topics in your state?

3. What are the so-called Baby Doe cases? Why are they so controversial?

B. Advanced Questions

1. Define the two classes of ethical systems, deontological and teleological, and give examples of each as they relate to the ethical dimensions of health care and health policy.

2. List three government agencies involved with new technology in the field of health care. State the function of each agency and which branch of government it is part of. Give an example of a current issue each agency is involved with.

3. Select a recent legal case involving nurses. Outline its history, explaining both sides of the argument, the strategies nurses took, and the final outcome. How might it affect other nurses? Examples of cases include *Sermchief* vs. *Gonzales;* pay equity cases; restrictions on nurse-midwifery practice in Washington, D.C.; other cases in your area.

4. Select a new technology. Discuss its ethical, legal, political, and economic ramifications. Interview a patient who is being treated or provider who is treating patients with this technology. What is the current status of third-party insurance coverage? What does the future hold for this technology in terms of demand, supply, cost, revision, and other aspects of use? Examples of possible technologies include organ transplants, artificial hearts, new medication such as cyclosporine, extracorporeal shock wave, lithotripsy, and magnetic resonance imaging.

VI. *Politics and Political Participation*

A. Basic Questions

    1. Give an example of an issue or situation in your professional life or clinical placement that demonstrates concepts of power and politics.

    2. State five basic principles that make for effective visiting and letter writing to legislators.

    3. What are three major legislative priorities identified by nurses or the state nurses' association in your state?

    4. Give examples of three coalitions, organizations, or special-interest groups that would be helpful to nursing in passing legislation for each of the items in question **A3** above.

B. Advanced Questions

    1. Refer to question **A3** above. Choose one item on the list. What are current strategies for enactment? What is the major opposition and why? What stage in the legislative process is it in? What will you personally do to be more actively involved with one of these issues?

    2. You are selected by a legislative committee to present testimony. Outline the process of preparing testimony. What do you need to know or do to be an expert witness?

    3. Select a partner. Together, role play a visit by a nurse to a federal, state, or county legislator or legislative staff person to lobby for a particular health care or nursing issue. Switch roles. Report on this experience.

VII. *Future Options*

A. Basic Questions

    1. What are health systems agencies? What is their function? What is a certificate of need?

2. Cite an example of health planning being done in either your clinical setting, a private organization, or a state or federal health agency or committee.

3. Select a nurse who is a leader in policy or a change agent in your facility or school. Describe three traits this person demonstrates that you believe contribute to her or his effectiveness.

B. Advanced Questions

1. What are health systems agencies (HSAs)? What are their advantages and disadvantages? Give an example of a recent decision taken by an HSA in your area. Who are the members of the HSA and how are they appointed? If possible, attend an HSA meeting and report to your colleagues.

2. Given these three factors to be considered in health planning—money, manpower, demand for health services—what type of planning would you recommend for your geographic or clinical area? How does the local situation compare in terms of these factors with the national scene? For each of the three factors, what are the specific constraints to be considered in establishing priorities? What data do you need to complete your health planning?

3. What strengths can you bring to the political process? What are your weaknesses and what is your plan over the next year to eliminate them? List specific activities and include an evaluation plan.

Answers to Exercises

I. Historical Evolution of Delivery of Health Care and Nursing

A. Basic Questions

1. There were many ways that Florence Nightingale exemplified the potential of nurses as influencers of public policy:

a. As a reformer of hospital care, she upgraded the quality of patient care by standardizing nursing care. She astutely made these standards and improvements acceptable practice in a system that was resistant to change and subject to the authority of military and public officials.

b. By upgrading the skills and knowledge required of nurses, Nightingale also advanced the status of women. Her professionalization of nursing and recruitment of well-educated women from higher economic and social classes upgraded the profession and its women members in the eyes of the public.

c. Nightingale extended nursing from acute hospital settings to the community. In so doing, she upgraded health care policies for the homebound and the public health of the community at large and dramatically changed the role of nursing.

d. Her public health work also included sanitation and efforts to improve community health conditions in general.

e. She strove to improve access to and quality of health care for all persons, regardless of their ability to pay.

f. Nightingale, as an advocate for nursing, sought better working conditions for nurses in all areas, such as pay, housing and time off. Her standards in this area eventually became accepted as hospital policy.

g. As an educator, Nightingale reformed educational policies for nursing by standardizing nursing education, establishing separate nursing educational programs, and recommending some form of certification (not merely registration) as a prerequisite to nursing practice.

2. Causes of the federal government's high health care bills: (1) growing number of elderly persons eligible for Medicare; (2) Medicare's previous reasonable-cost reimbursement method allowed for continually rising Medicare payments to the hospital; (3) advanced technology led to higher health care costs. In general, across the health care industry, spiraling health care costs were increasing three times faster than the gross national product; the federal government spent large amounts of money on entitlement and other programs, little of which was

picked up by the private sector and state and local governments.

3. The major justification for federal funding of nursing education is to increase the nation's supply of graduate-prepared nurses. This argument is based on the recommendations of the 1983 Institute of Medicine study entitled *Nursing and Nursing Education: Public Policies and Private Actions*: In this congressionally mandated study, it was stated that the previous critical shortage of nurses had abated and that nurses with master's and doctoral degrees were needed as educators, clinicians, administrators, and researchers. The study also recommended that more federal money be spent on nursing research and that nursing research be more closely integrated with the federal government's health care research activities.

B. Advanced Questions

1. Major focus of health care legislation in the past three decades: The 1960s were characterized by growth in domestic and social programs, emanating first from the Kennedy Administration and then from President Johnson's "Great Society." The latter included the Social Security legislation that established the Medicare and Medicaid programs. The Nurse Training Act was first passed in the mid-1960s, as a result of the federal government's commitment to provide health care for all and the ensuing need for more nurses and doctors and other health care professionals.

   The early 1970s continued the growth of the 1960s, but the rest of the 1970s were characterized by the federal government's recognition of the need to control rapidly rising health care costs, especially hospital costs. The government tried voluntary hospital cost-containment legislation, Professional Standard Review Organizations (PSROs), and the Tax Equity and Fiscal Responsibility Act as ways of monitoring Medicare costs. Congress also considered national health insurance and took an interest in health maintenance organizations as alternative ways of providing care and controlling cost.

   The 1980s will be known for enactment of Medicare's prospective payment system (PPS) for hospital reimbursement. This landmark legislation was considered necessary in order to control costs and alleviate the threatened insolvency of the Medicare trust fund. Even before the PPS was enacted, the Reagan administration had taken steps to cut health care costs and encourage the states and private sector to assume responsibility for health care programs that previously were mostly in the federal government's domain. In 1981, an Omnibus Reconciliation Act combined over twenty categorical programs into four block grants as a way of reducing costs. In the process, cuts were made in several health care programs. Many policy analysts say that one effect of the Reagan Administration's cuts was to decrease regulation while increasing competition and entrepreneurialism among health care providers. There is no doubt that the 1980s brought about an increase in competition and entrepreneurialism, plus greater diversification and a new role for proprietary health providers. There was greater linkage between business and health care and more emphasis on alternative delivery systems and ways to provide cost-effective health care in order to hold down health care costs and reduce the federal budget deficit.

2. Your answer should briefly summarize the major thoughts or ideas attributed to the thinker and explain how they were distinguishable from those of other major political thinkers of that time. The influence on American government should be shown by giving an example of a structure, process, or ideology that is part of our government and is in some way linked to this person's ideas. For purposes of this question, only the link need be shown: the way it came about is not important.

3. The two examples cited should give an idea of what is expected here. The answer should include three parts:

a. Identification of the clinical problem.

b. Specific policy-related knowledge that the student has now but lacked then. This could include a program, process, proposal, etc.

c. Link between **a** and **b** and how it could improve patient care.

Other possible examples: (a) terminally ill elderly patient eligible for reimbursement of hospice care under Medicare; (b) rehabilitation nurse caring for a patient who is discharged from the hospital still needing nursing care. If the nurse's state's law allows for direct third-party reimbursement for nursing care, the nurse could provide that care or refer the patient to a colleague.

II. Health Policy Analysis and Program Evaluation

A. Basic Questions

1. Nurses are well prepared to contribute to all phases of health care policy analysis.

a. Because of their first-hand experience and clinical expertise, nurses are particularly knowledgeable about health care delivery and, as a result, are able to help determine the scope of a policy problem. For instance, as providers of care to the elderly, nurses can give feedback to policy makers about the delivery and financing of long-term care. Nurses can provide information to help analysts and policy makers avoid suboptimization of policy problems (see "Key Concepts in Public Policy" at the beginning of this Workbook).

b. Nurses can provide clear information on criteria that may be used to determine a particular program's effectiveness and efficiency. For example, nurses delivering care can provide information useful for costing out nursing service; in turn, costing information can make a useful contribution to refinement of Medicare's prospective payment mechanisms.

c. Nurses can participate in discussing and determining the ethical criteria utilized in policy choice. For instance, nurses have valuable information on such issues as whether health care should be rationed and how to care for the terminally ill.

d. Nurses can also contribute by collecting data for program evaluation.

e. Nurses can play the role of "bellweather" by assessing feasibility of implementing a given identified policy in the current health care environment.

f. Nurses can prepare and deliver expert testimony and lobby on behalf of a particular policy or piece of legislation.

2. A bill may originate in either the Senate or House. After it is introduced, it is labeled with the name of the sponsors, then numbered, referred to the appropriate committee, and sent to the Government Printing Office so that copies can be made. If the President wants legislation to be considered by Congress, he must secure a Senate and/or House sponsor.

Most action on a bill takes place in committees, where all hearings are held and most amendments are introduced. Each committee has jurisdiction over certain subjects, and all measures affecting a particular area are referred to that committee. Membership on various committees is generally divided between the two major political parties in proportion to their total membership in the House or Senate.

When a bill reaches committee, it may be considered by the full committee or assigned by the chairman to a subcommittee for study and hearings. If a bill is assigned to a subcommittee, the subcommittee considers the bill and subsequently reports its recommendations and any proposed amendments to the full committee. In mark-up, a committee or subcommittee studies the bill, adds amendments to it, and decides whether to "report it out" for action or to "kill" the bill by not reporting it out. Many votes during mark-up are not recorded, and therefore legislators' votes are not released to the public. When a committee does send a bill to the floor, it also submits a written report that summarizes the legislation and includes committee views and interpretations of the bill.

In the House of Representatives, the

Rules Committee must assign a rule governing the time allowed for debate and the types of amendments that may be offered on the House floor. The amount of time granted for debate on a bill is controlled by the chairman and ranking minority member of the committee that handled the bill.

Under certain circumstances, the Speaker of the House may entertain a motion to "suspend the rules" in order to bring a bill or resolution directly to the House for consideration. The rules may be suspended only by an affirmative vote of two-thirds of the members voting, a quorum being present. This process is adopted in order to speed up the legislative process and is usually limited to noncontroversial bills.

In the Senate, a bill reported out of committee is placed directly on the Senate calendar. When general debate on a bill itself is concluded in either house, many separate votes may occur on various amendments before the entire bill is finally approved or rejected.

Although some legislation can be considered simultaneously by both houses, often a bill is passed in one house and then sent to the other for consideration. The second body may take one of several steps: (1) It may send the bill to the appropriate committee for consideration. (2) It may pass the bill as is, accepting the originating chamber's language. (3) It may reject the entire bill, advising the other house of its action. (4) It may produce its own version of the proposed legislation.

Often the second chamber makes only minor changes. If these are readily accepted by the first house, the bill then is routed directly to the President for signature. However, if the opposite chamber substantively alters the bill submitted to it, the measure is usually "sent to conference."

A conference committee undertakes to harmonize conflicting House and Senate versions of a bill. The presiding officers of the two houses select conference participants, known as conferees, from among members of the committees that handled the bills. Frequently the reconciliation of differences takes days or even weeks. When conferees do reach agreement, they submit to each house a conference report of their recommendations. Approval of the report by both houses constitutes approval of the compromise bill. If the conference committee is unable to reconcile all the differences in the bills, the issues in disagreement go back to both houses for consideration. If compromise between the two houses proves impossible, the bills are said to have "died" in conference.

After a bill has been passed by both the House and Senate, it is sent to the White House for the President's signature. If he does not sign it within ten days (Sundays excepted) and Congress is in session, the bill becomes law without his signature. If Congress is not in session, the President may *pocket veto* the bill (see Glossary).

The President may refuse to approve a bill and return it to the Congress with a message to the chamber that initiated the bill stating the reasons for his veto. If no further action is taken, the bill dies. Sometimes, however, Congress attempts to override the President's veto and thereby enact the bill. Congress may override a veto by a two-thirds vote of those legislators present at the time of the vote in each house. If the President's veto is overridden, the bill becomes law; otherwise it dies.

Nurses can influence the legislative process by proposing ideas for legislation to their representatives and providing feedback on bills already drafted. They can do this informally through letters and visits and through the more formal process of presenting testimony at committee hearings. They can also urge leaders in both houses to take prompt action in bringing a particular bill to the floor for a vote. At the critical point of a floor vote, they can make their recommendations to their legislators; finally, when the bill goes to the President for signing, nurses can contact the White House expressing their views.

3. The *Federal Register*, a document published every federal working day, is the government's official publication of

revisions in the code of federal regulations. It includes proposed rules and regulations and federal notices. Copies are obtained from the Superintendent of Documents (see Resource List), by going to the public library, or on a subscription basis ($300 per year).

In order to comment on a set of regulations, you need a copy of the most recent set of regulations as they appear in the *Code of Federal Regulations* (this is published once a year; same sources as above). Look in index to find out what other regulations were published on the topic in the recent past. You also must know the date the comment period ends, to whom to address the response, and the type of regulation (i.e., interim, final, proposed).

4. Congressional committees carry out the central functions of Congress. They process bills that have been introduced, hold hearings and mark up proposed legislation, investigate and identify the need for new legislation and for further research, and oversee the part of the executive branch that corresponds to the committee's jurisdiction (e.g., the Senate Labor and Human Resources Committee and the House Energy and Commerce Committee Subcommittee on Health are two of the many committees that oversee the Department of Health and Human Services).

Committee staff members draft legislation and deal with lobbyists. They carry out administrative, research, and public relations functions. Staff members are considered experts on the committee's area of jurisdiction and have considerable influence in determining the outcome of legislation because they make their recommendations directly to the committee chairperson. They may report to the chairperson of the committee or subcommittee or may have more general responsibilities to the committee as a whole, making their work less partisan in nature.

Special-interest groups represent organizations, industries, segments of the population (e.g., women, minorities, ethnic groups, the elderly), and geographic regions. They monitor and propose legislation to advance their causes. They may act either to defeat legislation perceived as harmful to the group or to propose and support legislation that would work to the group's advantage.

B. Advanced Questions

1. Three key criteria to be used in evaluating a program are *effectiveness*, *efficiency* and *equity*. A program's effectiveness focuses on whether its goals were achieved or there were any benefits received from the program. Efficiency focuses on whether the benefits received from the program outweigh the resources (costs) invested. Equity deals with the criterion of fairness. To evaluate the equity of a program, one considers the morality of the actions taken and asks whether the program benefitted large numbers of people or focused only on a small segment of the population. In addition, were any mechanisms set in place that could prevent entry into the program by some groups but not by others? Principles that can assist in determining fairness include the *utilitarian principle* and *Pareto optimality*. The utilitarian principle is concerned with which policy or program maximizes the sum of utility (units of pleasure) in society. A program is said to be Pareto optimal when, as a result of the program, no one person is better or worse off than another.

The objectives of the federal government's health maintenance organization program are to (1) provide financial assistance for the start-up and operation of HMOs; (2) develop standards of care; and (3) promote access to HMOs by requiring employers who offer health insurance to offer an HMO option to their employees.

Questions one might ask about this program that relate to the criteria of effectiveness, efficiency, and equity include:

Effectiveness

—Has financial aid resulted in expansion of HMOs?
—Are the HMOs that have received financial assistance viable and

successful?

—How effective have the standards of care been in improving quality of care?

Efficiency

—Are there more ways of securing development capital than federal funds (e.g., private-sector funds such as venture capital, sale of stock)?

Equity

—Has the program provided greater access to HMOs? For example, have the unemployed been benefitted?

2. Problems can be prioritized simply by individual preference; however, it is preferable to have some rationale for policy decisions. Whatever problems you consider, the decision to give priority to one program over another should be based on some accepted method of policy inquiry. Three traditional policy inquiry approaches are behaviorism, economic analysis, and interpretive analysis.

    Behaviorism is a doctrine that states that data consist exclusively of observable evidence. In other words, one can study and seek for causes among only those phenomena that can be seen directly. Behaviorists are concerned with empirical evidence and use the scientific method to test out experimental hypotheses.

    The *economic* approach employs rationality as its model, defining a rational being as one who maximizes expected satisfaction. This approach incorporates both empirical and normative concerns. Strategies such as benefit–cost analysis can be used to weigh the benefits received from one program against the costs invested in that program. Comparisons between programs can then be used to determine which program yields more benefits for the costs incurred. The normative economic concerns relate to the justification of economic decisions. Models such as utilitarianism and Pareto optimality provide rules to follow (see question **1** above).

    The *interpretive* approach is an-

tagonistic to positivism (use of the scientific method and sole dependence on reason) and uses the participant-observer method to determine patterns of behavior. The product of a study carried out by means of this approach is a verbal description of the subject that seeks to find meaning in phenomena and the relationships among them.

In example **a**, taking an economic approach, several factors are important in deciding which prenatal intervention will most effectively decrease the demand for high-cost newborn intensive care services. If the choices are maternal nutrition programs, prenatal care targetted for adolescent mothers, or outreach to certain low socioeconomic populations, the cost–benefit analysis of each approach would include the immediate costs of implementing the program as well as the long-term savings to the agency, the patient, and society because of the contributions good prenatal care can make in alleviating the need for high-tech interventions and preventing congenital illnesses. Program implementation costs vary depending on the program's scope, duration, population size, personnel, and the availability of funding. These are the types of issues that should be explained in detail in your answer.

Other factors to consider are the long-term benefits to the provider and patient, marketing and public relations considerations, and to what extent the agency must conduct a program because of public relations benefits that will mean greater business for or utilization of the agency in the long run. Your answer should include discussion of how some of these areas would be assessed. Whenever possible, relate your answer to the demographics and demand for health care in your particular geographic area.

3. Some of the common reasons that the findings of program evaluation do not affect policy implementation include:

a. The data may be incomplete, not presented in a timely fashion, or documented in such a way that the results have no relationship to the issues or program objectives. The findings may also have a potentially negative influence on the longetivity of the program or its administrative participants.

b. The participants in the evaluation may not be clear on the scope or the intent of the evaluation and therefore may not carry out a complete or accurate study. The evaluators may also focus on only certain aspects of the evaluation, which may or may not relate to the intended policy. The program's administration may choose not to validate the findings, especially if they are not in line with their goals.

c. Politics, both internal and external, may hinder the effectiveness of an evaluation. If the political climate is contrary to the findings, the results of the evaluation may be summarized in a fashion that is in alignment with the political objectives, they may be delayed in transit to key decision makers, or they may never be made known.

III. Politics and Economics of Health Care Financing

A. Basic Questions

1. Several agencies can be cited in answering this question.

    The Health Care Financing Administration (HCFA) within the Department of Health and Human Services (DHHS) is responsible for the Medicare and Medicaid programs. Its nearly $100 billion annual budget makes it very important for health care financing.

    Another example is the Office of Management and Budget within the White House. This agency makes recommendations to the President regarding the federal budget and funding of all federal programs, including health care.

    Other agencies are: (1) the Congressional Budget Office (CBO), which provides analysis of budget proposals, including those affecting health care, to Congress; and (2) the Health Resources and Services Administration (HRSA) within the Public Health Service (PHS), which also plays a role in the allocation of federal funds for health care, especially health manpower programs and the health care delivery programs for target populations (such as the Indian Health Services). Other possibilities are the Office of Technology Assessment, the General Accounting Office, and the Office of the Inspector General within DHHS.

2. Medicare's previous reasonable-cost reimbursement system reimbursed hospitals according to the costs they submitted to the federal government, based on Medicare's definition of reasonable cost. Under prospective payment, hospitals are paid a fixed amount for a Medicare patient's hospitalization, based on the assignment of that patient to a particular diagnosis related group (DRG). The hospital is reimbursed only one rate per DRG, no matter what the costs to the hospital are. If the hospitalization costs more than the DRG reimbursement rate, then the hospital must make up the difference. Hospitals now have more of an incentive to hold down costs than they did under the cost-based system. Under that system, although payments were limited, in general, hospitals received payments covering a significant proportion of their incurred costs.

3. An authorization bill, a prerequisite for an appropriations bill, is legislation enacted by Congress establishing program policies and parameters and establishing a budget limit for the programs. Once an authorization bill is passed, Congress must pass yearly appropriations legislation to determine the actual amount of funds that will be available for the authorized program. Under the Constitution, the House initiates all appropriations bills.

4. No matter which DRG is chosen, the basic premise is the same. That is, there is a wide range of utilization of nursing resources within a DRG. The differences are primarily due to severity of illness,

need for psychosocial support, patient education, counseling, discharge planning, and other nursing measures not accounted for within the DRG payment. For example, two diabetic patients (DRG 294) admitted with ketoacidosis might require different nursing resources. A patient who has a good understanding of his illness, strong family support, expertise in blood glucose monitoring, and maintains a steady diet and exercise regime will not require as much nursing care as another patient who has had very poor control, has never learned to care for himself, and does not speak English very well.

Similar differences in nursing care can be found for each of the DRGs listed.

5a. Medicare is a federal entitlement program for individuals who have employment covered by Social Security. These people automatically become eligible for Medicare upon reaching age 65. It also covers disabled individuals and those with end stage renal disease. For patients in the latter categories, age is not a factor. Medicaid provides medical assistance to individuals in certain categories through a program financed by both federal and state funds. Eligibility is limited to those who are aged, blind, disabled, or enrolled in AFDC (Aid to Families with Dependent Children) programs. Although there is federal legislation establishing the parameters of the Medicaid program, each state is responsible for the administration of its Medicaid program and for establishing the specific income eligibility criteria for its enrollees.

5b. Medicare Part A provides coverage for institutional care, including acute hospital care. It is financed through Social Security payroll taxes. Medicare Part B provides coverage for physicians' fees, other professional services, and medical supplies. Enrollment is voluntary, and the program is financed by premium payments and federal general revenues.

5c. The Tax Equity and Fiscal Responsibility Act (TEFRA) of 1982 is legislation that preceded Medicare's prospective pay-

ment system. For the first time, it established a limit, per case or per admission, on the amount that Medicare would reimburse hospitals under Part A of Medicare. It also directed Congress to devise a prospective payment system for Medicare by 1983.

B. Advanced Questions

1. The following is an outline of the major points of the federal budget process, incorporating the balanced-budget legislation enacted by Congress in December 1985. This schedule applies to the fiscal years 1987-1991, and therefore was initiated in calendar year 1986.

January - February: The President submits his budget for the next fiscal year, which begins Oct. 1, to Congress. Any automatic cost-of-living increase scheduled to take effect on Jan. 1 would be deferred until it is determined that automatic spending cuts are not necessary. If that is the case, the cost of living increases would be restored retroactive to Jan. 1.

April 15: Congress is supposed to complete action on the budget resolution for the next fiscal year, based on the recommendations of the budget committee.

June 15: Congress is supposed to approve the deficit reduction bill needed to impose much of the savings proposed in the budget resolution:

June 30: The House is to have finished all its appropriations bills, where additional savings to reduce the deficit would be made. There is no deadline for the Senate.

August 15: The OMB and the CBO do their deficit estimates based on completed budget action to date.

August 20: OMB and CBO send report to General Accounting Office.

August 25: The automatic spending cut order, if the deficit ceiling is breached, is sent to the President.

September 1: The President issues the automatic spending cut order, with 50 percent of the total cuts taken from the military budget and 50 percent cut from the nonmilitary programs.

October 1: The fiscal year begins and the automatic spending cuts take effect.

October 5: OMB and CBO issue final deficit projection report to reflect final congressional action to reduce the deficit. The report goes to the GAO.

October 10: The revised GAO report goes to the President.

October 15: The final order for automatic spending cuts, based on the revisions, goes into effect.

2. Competition operates on the principle that the forces of supply and demand in the marketplace will interact so as to ensure that resources are allocated most efficiently. It is a more open system than one based on regulation, under which the price, quality, and utilization of goods, in this case, health care services, are defined by the government. A regulatory-oriented system requires all participants to adhere to a uniform standard of practice, defined by the government, and allows less innovation than a competitively oriented system.

There are no absolute right or wrong answers in discussing ways that both competition and regulation can be ascribed to Medicare's prospective payment system. Some analysts believe that the Reagan Administration's prospective payment system has created a health care environment that is more regulatory than ever before, especially if one considers the methods for establishing DRG prices and the tighter utilization review and quality assurance activities to be carried out by peer review organizations. Others say that the Reagan administration, in true Republican tradition, has implemented prospective payment in order to create a more competitive health care marketplace in which efficiencies in management, marketing, and financing can be rewarded. This would replace the previous system, which had little incentive for competitive practices and efficiencies in operation.

In answering this question, you need not ascribe to only one point of view. However, you should give concrete examples to substantiate your arguments and demonstrate clarity of thought.

3. In interviewing a nurse administrator in order to ascertain what her greatest challenges have been under DRGs, be sure to obtain concrete examples. For example, managing a budget or cutting costs are not sufficient answers. Determine specifically which aspects of budget management have presented problems, what dilemmas she has faced in attempting to resolve these problems, and what conflicts have occurred between different interest groups within the hospital. If cutting costs was an issue, try to determine who decides which costs can be cut and the degree of autonomy that the administrator has in her decisions. To find this out, you would also need to have an overall sense of the organization of the hospital and where this administrator fits within the structure.

Students should also find out what new personal challenges DRGs have presented to the nursing administrator (in terms of professional or career development). The answer should include some explanation of how this person places priority on the interests of her staff, patients, and the agency and a discussion of how much these priorities vary from issue to issue. Again, be sure to elicit concrete examples.

4. This is another question without right or wrong answers. Your answers will reflect your particular interests and what you see as the most important challenges of the health care system today. The point is that for each audience, the focus must change in order to address the issues that are of particular concern for them. For example, a nursing group needs to understand that DRGs do not take into account variations in nursing costs. It is also important for them to realize that with stiffer competition and a surplus of physicians, there are opportunities for them to market their cost-effective services, while there is a simultaneous need to maintain a tight vigilance on state legislative activities in order to circumvent efforts, spearheaded primarily by physicians, to restrict nurses' scope of practice and opportunities for direct third-party reimbursement.

Nurses will have to be made cognizant of the political and economic forces at play in community health care, which has historically been nurses' domain. The need to market nursing services here and to recognize the political forces that affect nurses' ability to maintain their stake in this sector is sharper than ever before. These are just a few examples of items to be considered in addressing a nursing audience on this topic.

In contrast, a consumer audience will need basic education about the health care system in general. It will be helpful for them to have basic background information about prospective payment, emphasizing the problems it poses for them in terms of quality of care, coordination of care, and their need to be informed and assertive in their role as purchasers of care (e.g., seeking second opinions, alternative providers, etc.). Consumers should be shown that they have options and what these options are. In other words, the emphasis for the consumer audience will be on teaching them to help themselves.

The elderly will be particularly concerned about Medicare, long-term care, chronic illness, and coordination of social needs with medical needs. Like the consumer group, they need to hear about the range of options available to them, with an emphasis on the concerns of the elderly, such as day care, education concerning their medications and diseases, and identification of resources in the community available to them. Consumer groups specifically serving the elderly, such as AARP and the Grey Panthers, should be described as resources and as advocates of the elderly in the politics and economics of health care delivery.

IV. Alternative Delivery Systems: Issues and Problems

A. Basic Questions

1. See Glossary for definitions of these terms.

2. Each of these alternative delivery systems provides the consumer with choices and advantages in terms of cost, style, and access to health care services. HMOs do not charge a fee for each

service delivered, and patients can receive a wide range of services at a lower cost than would obtain with a private physician. The enrollment fee for the HMO covers the costs of the HMO services. Patients enrolled in HMOs receive comprehensive care with an emphasis on prevention, because of the HMO's incentive to reduce acute-care and emergency-room visits and hospitalizations. When patients need referral to a specialist, problems of coordination are minimized because the specialists are usually participating physicians in the HMO.

Preferred provider organizations offer the consumer many of the same advantages as HMOs: incentives to prevent costly acute-care visits and coverage of routine office visits. PPOs often pass cost savings on to the consumer in the form of lower premiums. Compared to HMOs, PPOs usually offer the patient a wider choice of alternative providers.

The major advantages of urgent care centers are their location and price, compared to more traditional hospital emergency-room services.

Birthing centers offer patients an informal environment specifically designed for healthy deliveries, with an emphasis on family participation. In addition, birthing centers often offer comprehensive packages that cost less than the more traditional arrangements offered by hospitals. Birthing centers are inclined to use nurse-midwives and to minimize the impersonal atmospheres of hospital labor and delivery rooms.

3. For this question, students should contact their state nurses' association or other appropriate resources. If legislation has been enacted, obtain a copy of the bill. If regulations have been issued, review them. Furthermore, if there is proposed legislation for any specialty nursing group, such as nurse-midwives or nurse practitioners, then obtain copies of those bills if possible, or at least familiarize yourself with the basic points of the legislation. By answering this question, you should also learn about some of the politics involved in obtain-

ing direct third-party reimbursement for nurses in your state.

B. Advanced

1. *Vertical integration* is an economic term referring to expansion across diverse lines of production, resulting in movement into various related (in this case, health care) activities. Through vertical integration, a broad range of services can be offered under the management of one company or corporation. A vertically integrated facility can offer a range of services, beginning with the patient's initial contact with an emergency room or clinic, and continuing through hospitalization and the subsequent discharge needs of skilled nursing care, home care, or hospice. Each hospital may choose to integrate a different range of services, depending on which services are in greatest demand and which will prove to be most profitable. As a result of DRGs, there has been an increased use of vertical integration as a management strategy to increase admissions and revenues—two areas that are of particular concern to hospital administrators under prospective payment. Vertical integration is a means hospitals can use to offset declining revenues; it also enables hospitals to maintain tighter control of the patient for a broader range of health care services, including acute care and well visits. Vertical integration can also apply to nonprofit facilities and sole community hospitals.

National Medical Enterprises (NME) and Humana are often cited as examples of companies with vertical integration. NME has begun to build medical campuses where a variety of health care facilities are provided in one location. A campus might include physicians' offices, skilled nursing facility, acute-care hospital, mental health center, and other health care facilities. Humana has diversified to include skilled nursing care, acute care, ambulatory care, outreach programs, and high-tech tertiary care, such as the heart transplantation program.

There are two types of *horizontal integration*. One refers to the engaging in of activities that were not previously performed and are in a related, but not the same, line of production. This would include hospitals that expand their food services beyond the hospital's needs and begin to contract with Meals on Wheels programs in the community to provide food services, or hospitals that operate a hotel or residential facility for patients' families and other general nonmedical purposes.

The second form of horizontal integration refers to broadening of essentially the same activities within the same or related market by means of mergers and acquisitions. These multiistitutional arrangements offer hospitals the advantages of efficiency, economies of scale, and greater access to capital. In addition to the traditional types of merges, hospitals are also forming horizontal arrangements that include hospital consortia, affiliates, alliances, and joint ventures.

The best-known example of horizontal integration in the health care industry is the proprietary chains. The largest single acquisition of a hospital company by another hospital company occurred when, in 1981, Hospital Corporation of America took over Hospital Affiliates International. Another well-known merger was the 1979 takeover by Humana of American Medicorp. Horizontal integration can also apply to nonprofit hospital chains, such as Sisters of Mercy hospitals, which are acquiring many hospitals located primarily in the west. In answering this question, students are encouraged to give examples of horizontal or vertical integration that have occurred within their immediate vicinity.

2. You may select any legislative proposal, from the federal, state, or county level, that promotes an alternative health care delivery system. Resources available include state and national nursing organizations, as well as periodicals and newsletters published by nursing and other health care organizations. You can also contact legislative staff members or their representatives to obtain information on the most recent legislative initiatives.

In researching the pros and cons of the bill, interview legislators and special-interest groups working for and against it in order to get a sense of the politics involved and the bill's chances of enactment.

Implications for nursing should include the ways the bill could positively affect nursing and promote access to nursing care, as well as challenges and potential obstacles it could present for the profession.

3. There are, of course, many examples of patients whom nurses have cared for who have experienced the fragmentation of the health care delivery system. Usually, these patients have complex or chronic illnesses, and they often fall at the very beginning and end of the age spectrum.

For example, perinatal care is often fragmented, with prenatal care being offered in one place, labor and delivery in another, and postpartum care for the mother and child in yet a third. Birthing centers that offer all the services together, or HMOs, which also provide comprehensive packages and have primary nurse practitioners or physicians as coordinators of care, help alleviate these problems.

As another example, case management poses a special challenge for the elderly and those with chronic illnesses. In these instances, case management refers to coordination of care and guiding the patient to the appropriate resources. Nurses are in a prime position to be case managers because of their appreciation of the full range of a patient's physical, emotional, and social needs. HMOs and other vertically integrated facilities help to alleviate these problems, as does the use of a gatekeeper, such as a nurse, to reduce unnecessary and costly duplication of health care services.

Your answer should include a brief explanation of the patient's chief complaint, history, and management problem, stating specifically what services the patient received and how fragmentation was a problem. For solutions, alternative use of existing resources or innovative ways of developing new

resources are acceptable answers.

4. This exercise requires that you obtain the names of people to interview at a third-party payer and an employer in the community and interview both, either by phone or in person. Often companies have public relations or communications staff who can answer questions or direct you to the appropriate person. You should not limit yourself to the questions listed here; rather, use them as a starting point. Someone, either teacher or student, should take responsibility for coordinating the contacts so that a wide range of companies are included and duplication is avoided. It would be interesting for some students to present their findings to the class, so that students can appreciate the diversity of concerns in the community.

Before conducting the interview, be sure to learn about the company. Obtain a copy of the annual report or a description of the benefit package they offer their employers or their customers. Prepare your questions in advance, and ask a classmate to accompany you if you prefer. Be sure to follow up your interview with a thank-you note. Also, assure the person you interview that the information is for a class only and will not be published or released in any form.

After answering this question, you should have a sense of the areas of mutual concern and of conflict between third-party payers and employers. For example, does the employer want certain services included in the benefits package that the insurer does not? Who is responsible for holding down health care costs, and how?

V. Technological, Legal, and Ethical Dimensions of Health Care

A. Basic Questions

1. Some of the agencies that can be included in the answer to this question are:

a. Office of Technology Assessment (OTA), which provides information and analyses to Congress on the political, physical, economic, and social effects of technological applications. For further information and a list of publications, contact the Office of Technology Assessment, U.S. Congress, Washington,

The National Center for Health Services Research and Health Care Technology Assessment is located within the Public Health Service of the Department of Health and Human Services (DHHS). It conducts studies on the measurement of health status, the organization and delivery of health services (especially for long-term care), health care policy for Medicare, state and local health programs, and the safety and effectiveness of new medical technologies with regard to Medicare coverage. For further information, contact NCHSR-HCTA, 5600 Fishers Lane, Rockville, MD 20857.

The Food and Drug Administration (FDA) is located within the PHS, DHHS. Its function is to conduct research and develop standards for the safety, quality, and effectiveness of food and drug products and medical devices. For further information, contact Food and Drug Administration, 5600 Fishers Lane, Rockville, MD 20857.

This list is not meant to be finite. It represents the major federal agencies involved with health care technology. Other agencies include the National Institute for Occupational Safety and Health (NIOSH), the National Science Foundation, and the Prospective Payment Assessment Commission (ProPAC).

2. To answer this question, you can select several types of nursing legislation that pertain to nursing practice. Some of the most important ones are nurse practice acts, legislation on direct third-party reimbursement, and legislation on scope of practice for specialty groups, such as nurse practitioners and nurse-midwives. Scope of practice could also include prescription-writing privileges. Some states also have legislation on continuing education as a requirement for licensure. To obtain information about the laws on these topics in a particular state, contact the state nurses' association or state board of nursing.

3. Baby Doe cases are cases of newborns who are born with severe disabilities or handicaps and for whom the decision must be made whether to carry out life-sustaining activities. These infants have received attention because of two landmark cases that led to the federal government's involvement in establishing criteria for their care. As a result, legislation has been enacted and regulations promulgated to define the role of the government and of health care providers in caring for these children. These cases have raised controversy among special interest groups representing right-to-life interests, the handicapped, health care practitioners, and the government. (See Case Study 1.)

B. Advanced Questions

1. *Deontological* ethical systems are based on the discovery and confirmation of moral rules that govern the resolution of an ethical dilemma. Deontological theory holds that an action is right if it accords with a moral rule and wrong if it violates it. Deontologists judge the morality of an action not by its consequences but by what kind of action it is: an action is right not necessarily because it brings about good consequences but because it satisfies the requirements of a supreme principle of duty. Theological ethical systems make up this class. Under such a system, one might act to preserve life (a supreme principle) without considering the consequences for the patient. *Teleological* ethical systems focus on efficiency and utility. The "greatest good" is the overriding concern. Examples of this kind of system include:

a. Utilitarianism: a normative ethical system that holds that an action is morally right either because it brings about good consequences or it is of such a kind that, if everyone did it, would have good consequences. The underlying concept is utility, or usefulness. This system comes into play in cases where there is conflict between general welfare and individual patients' welfare.

b. Justice as fairness: under this system,

one considers rules and actions from the standpoint of the least advantaged in society. For example, under this system one would hold that the indigent population should not be denied entry into the Medicaid program based on an income test.

2. See basic question **A1** above. Reports recently published by OTA include *Medical Technology and the Costs of the Medicare Program, Managing the Nation's Commercial High-Level Radioactive Waste,* and *Blood Policy and Technology.* A report entitled *Nurse Practitioners, Certified Nurse Midwives, and Physician Assistants: Quality, Access, Economic and Payment Issues* is in progress. For a more complete listing of OTA reports, contact the OTA office.

    The FDA has approved every new drug, food additive, or cosmetic product put on the market, such as acyclovir, aspartame, human growth hormone, and food dyes, to name just a few. It has also been involved with product labeling, product recall, and research into medical devices such as cardiac pacemakers, magnetic resonance imaging, and the artificial heart

    The NCHSR-HCTA conducts the National Health Care Expenditures Study (NHCES), which provides estimates of coverage by private health insurance and public programs, as well as patterns of health care use and expenditures. Separate publications from this study include: *NHCES Data Preview 1: Who are the Uninsured?* (PHS 80-3276) and *NHCES Data Preview 22: Nonphysician Health Care Providers: Use of Ambulatory Services, Expenditures, and Sources of Payment* (PHS 85-3394). Examples of NCHSR-HCTA research regarding technology and Medicare coverage are a study of percutaneous ultrasound procedures for treatment of kidney stones and a study of magnetic resonance imaging, both done in 1985.

3. One case that can be cited is the controversy in the District of Columbia over expanded clinical privileges for nurses. On October 4, 1983, the District of Columbia became the first United States jurisdiction to pass a comprehensive

clinical privileges bill that prohibits hospitals and other licensed health care facilities from denying clinical privileges (including admitting privileges) and staff membership to five types of nonphysician providers: nurse anesthetists, nurse practitioners, nurse-midwives, psychologists, and podiatrists. The legislation makes it unlawful for a D.C. hospital to prevent any of the five providers, on a classwide basis, from practicing in its facility.

But for nurses in independent practice, such as Rene Smit, a certified nurse-midwife (CNM) who was employed by Washington Hospital Center as a labor and delivery nurse and who has a private nurse-midwifery practice, there are obstacles to practice. Smit was the first to attempt to exercise admitting privileges after the legislation was passed, and she met with opposition from the hospital's administrators. In June 1984 she applied for clinical privileges. They were granted, with the stipulation that a physician be present for labor and delivery once the woman had dilated beyond six centimeters. This limiting arrangement ran counter to what Smit and her attorney, who also works with the D.C. Nurses' Association (DCNA), considered the intent of the statute. The hospital's restrictions both called Smit's expertise into question and cost patients money—they must pay those back-up physicians.

D.C nurses rallied to Smit's and other nurses' sides by obtaining representation on committees charged with making recommendations for proposed regulations and providing input to the D.C. Department of Human Services. They also obtained the support of consumer groups in lobbying the government to show that limitations placed on nursing practice were in violation of the original clinical privileges statute. Smit and her attorney also officially requested that the corporation counsel, which is the equivalent of the state attorney general in the District of Columbia, investigate and prosecute this violation of the statute. Eventually, Smit set up her own fee-for-service practice, even though the hospital did not relent on the limitations it imposed on her practice.

Organized medicine's attempt to place restraints on expanded nursing practice is complicated by the fact that the D.C. nurse practice act lacked an updated definition of nursing practice, especially expanded practice. Nurses in the District have been working on revising their practice act to keep up with changing nursing and health care trends. In the process, they have run into serious obstacles, because the nurse practice act proposed by the D.C. legislators was very restrictive. It addressed expanded practice for only the three specialty nursing groups included in the clinical privileges legislation, omitting other groups, such as psychiatric nurses and clinical specialists. It also required protocols and severely limiting provisions for collaboration between physicians and nurses and informed consent for patients treated by CNMs.

Nurses testified against the nurse practice act legislation at hearings held on the bill. They also got other groups, such as the National Organization for Women, the Grey Panthers, and other consumer health activists to support their position. When the bill was marked up, many of the recommendations of the DCNA regarding collaboration and informed consent were added as amendments.

However, from the nurses' perspective the bill was still too restrictive, in terms of both nurse anesthetist practice and its references to medical practice acts as they pertained to nursing. DCNA was working to amend these areas before final enactment of the bill.

D.C. nurses are fighting in the legislative and regulatory arenas to uphold both the intent of the clinical privileges bill and their legitimate rights to survive and thrive as independent practitioners in the District of Columbia. This case calls to mind threats to nursing autonomy and professionalism across the country. Many groups of nurses are attempting to obtain clinical privileges and some have been successful. This case illustrates that even when clinical privileges are won there may still be opposition to independent practice,

expecially as the surplus of physicians increases. Whatever success the DCNA has achieved, it is the result of hard work, careful strategizing, and the extraordinary unity displayed within the nursing community, which formed the basis for liaison with other groups.

Whichever case you cite in answering this question, it should be presented in a format similar to this one.

4. Once the technology has been selected, do background reading: review of the recent medical and nursing literature as well as articles from the popular press. In planning for the interview, prepare questions suitable for the person being interviewed. The purpose of the interview should be to elicit opinion and first-hand experiences, rather than background information, which you should have obtained from you reading. For example, in interviewing a patient, you might ask how he decided to receive the treatment, how much it costs, who is paying for it, what he was told about the risks and benefits, who opposed the treatment and why, and who was in favor of it and why. Similar questions should be asked of the provider.

VI. Politics and Political Participation

A. Basic Questions

1. The example should describe the use of power to influence situations or people. Use of power implies the ability to make happen what we want to have happen. The discussion might include the different types of power, including *expert power* (having expertise in a particular area), *information power* (possessing information that another needs or wants), *reward* or *coercive power* (being able to provide or take away what another wants or values) and *referent power* (mutual trust and affection leading to influence). *Politics* is the use of power by individuals or interest groups. Politics can occur within organizations or in the public arena and can take on aspects of both positive manipulation (direct strategies such as lobbying for one's cause) and negative manipulation (indirect strategies such as passive-aggressive behavior or entrapment).

The example can be a situation that relates to organizational life, patient care, colleagial interaction, or activities in the public arena, such as activities within the professional association or interest groups.

2. See D. Mason & S. Talbott, *Political Action Handbook for Nurses* (Menlo Park, CA: Addison-Wesley, 1985), Chapter 29. Five basic principles are:

a. Always identify yourself as a nurse.

b. Prepare in advance: know how the legislator stands on the issue and be familiar with his or her political orientation (party affiliation, committees, assignments), and know how professional nursing organizations stand on the issue.

c. Be clear about what your opinion is and what you want the legislator to do.

d. If possible, send a brief fact sheet on the issue.

e. Follow up with a thank-you note and any additional information requested by the legislator.

3. Legislative priorities can be identified informally through feedback from nurses who are involved in activities that have a potential for legislative involvement (e.g., third-party reimbursement for nurses in extended practice) or formally through resolutions passed by the membership of the state nurses' association. Major legislative priorities might include:

a. Third-party reimbursement for nurses in expanded practice.

b. Modifications to the nurse practice act.

c. Family planning.

d. Health care cost containment.

e. State health planning.

f. Air and water quality.

4. Examples for several of the items in question **A3** include:

a. Third-party reimbursement for nurses: the state nurses' association, the nurse practitioner special-interest group, the state business coalition, and special-

interest groups that would utilize services of a nurse practitioner, such as the Grey Panthers, the American Association of Retired Persons, or the PTA.

b. Health care cost containment: the above groups would be helpful in this area as well, especially if one emphasized nursing's role in providing cost-effective care. In addition, the local hospital association, nurse executives' associations, and other health care specialty organizations would support the need for cost containment.

c. Air and water quality: local consumer groups would provide testimony that they desire a certain level of water quality. Environmental groups, such as the Sierra Club, also work in this area.

B. Advanced Questions

1. Answers will vary, but they should take the form of a case study, including background information and statement of the major issue involved. Be specific in stating your involvement with the issue.

2. See Mason and Talbott, *Political Action Handbook for Nurses*, Chapter 29. The main steps include the following:

a. Become familiar with the jurisdiction of legislative committees, their subcommittees, and their membership.

b. Find out the ground rules applicable to the hearing (e.g., time limitations, length of testimony, number of copies of printed testimony needed, deadline for submitting advance copies of testimony, etc.). Prepare testimony in accordance with the ground rules and in agreement with approved policies of your parent organization.

c. If you are not going to testify yourself, select a witness knowledgeable in the subject area.

d. Draft the written testimony first. Include a description of your organization, its membership, and why the hearings are important to its activities. In the body of the testimony, be sure to document your assertions with recent data.

e. Speak spontaneously whenever possible. This is always more effective than reading from a written text.

f. If possible, contact a committee staff member to suggest questions or to review the committee's questions in advance of the hearing.

g. Follow up after the hearing by promptly submitting any additional information requested.

3. Refer back to question **A2** above. The person playing the nurse should have a particular issue in mind to talk about. The person playing the legislator should have a particular person in mind and be familiar with his opinions. When the partners switch roles, the new "legislator" may impersonate a different person.

VII. Future Options

A. Basic Questions

1. See Glossary.

2. For your clinical setting, contact the hospital administrator or director of nursing. To find out about health planning being done by a private organization or state or federal agency, you might contact the state or national nursing, medical, or hospital associations; the local or state health department; or the American Public Health Association in Washington, D.C., or a state or local affiliate; or a staff person for a legislator on a key congressional health committee.

3. Answers will vary. Be sure to give examples of how the person demonstrates the traits you select.

B. Advanced Questions

1. See question **A1** above. Criticisms of HSAs, including those from the Reagan administration, focus on the regulatory burden they place on state and local governments, with no documentation that the effort put into their operations actually saves money in the long run. HSAs also run counter to the Reagan administration's competitive orientation. Some question whether the consumer participation in HSAs has been, or ever can be, fully effective. Others complain that there are too many conflicts of interest among HSA board members and that it is not fitting that the same people responsible for planning and monitoring health care are also the regulators and, in some cases, the providers and purchasers of care. It has also been argued that changes in the way both public and private programs purchase health care have resulted in restraints in capital investment that are as restrictive as or more restrictive than certificate of need (CON) programs have been, thus mitigating the need for CONs and HSAs.

Those in favor of maintaining the HSAs question if the medical marketplace, left to its own devices, would adequately monitor health planning and the purchasing of new equipment. They fear that without HSAs, there could be uncontrolled investment in new products, which could result in an unnecessary rise in hospital costs. Those in favor of maintaining HSAs also claim that with rising health care costs, we cannot afford not to have in place a system for planning and controlling these costs. They say that the program can be revised, so as to provide a greater flexibility to state and local health planning agencies, and that the need to prevent unnecessary and duplicative expansion of health services is still grave enough to justify their (HSAs) existence.

Congress is now reconsidering the role and existence of HSAs as part of the larger issue of whether the federal government should have a role in local health planning. The wider question, of course, is how and under what auspices local areawide health planning is to be carried out. Be sure to include recent developments in your answer.

In order to contact an HSA in your area, or ascertain if one exists, contact an administrator of a local hospital or a hospital health planning staff member or a state or local health department. Before attending an HSA meeting, it will be helpful to contact the HSA staff and inform them that you will be present.

2. Answers will vary depending on state and local situations. National priorities all point to a depleted federal budget and budget deficit. Hence funding for health care programs is tight, and money for new programs is particularly difficult to obtain. The federal government has identified certain priority spending areas, based on demographics and other social factors. Some of these are geriatrics, disease prevention, long-term care, and improving access to care for underserved populations. The federal government has granted most health programs little or no increases in funding in recent years.

Funding of health professions education is no longer a high priority for the federal government now that the critical shortage of these personnel has abated. For nursing, the government recognizes the need for graduate-prepared nurses and for federal funding of nursing research, largely because of the recommendation of the 1983 Institute of Medicine Report, *Nursing and Nursing Education: Public Policies and Private Actions*. Additional documentation on the supply and demand of registered nurses is available in the *Report to the President and the Congress on the Status of Health Personnel in the United States*. This document, published every few years, reports on many health professions and in recent reports has pointed to the importance of baccalaureate and master's prepared nurses, especially to meet community, long-term, and critical-care needs. The most recent report was completed in May 1984 and the next one is in progress, due to be completed in 1986. State health departments often issue similar types of reports on a state's need for nursing personnel, depending on the state's health planning needs.
ning needs.

To complete this exercise, you should be knowledgeable about at least one federal government report on nursing personnel in addition to the IOM study and the report to Congress. Then, obtain information about local planning priorities by contacting health planners and providers in your area.

3. Answers will vary. Be specific about strengths and weaknesses and give examples of how they affect your ability to participate. Be sure to include deadlines for meeting goals.

Case Studies

INTRODUCTION

The purpose of the following Case Studies is to encourage you to develop and use analytical thought processes. Use of these and other Case Studies, in class, individually, or with small groups of colleagues, will help you sharpen your skills in situation assessment, problem diagnosis, evaluation of alternative courses of action, and formulation of action plans.

Ideally case studies should be presented for group discussion and analysis. First, the group should identify the key points about the case. Then, the group should discuss alternative courses of action and recommendations for specific actions.

To prepare for class discussion, read through the case at least three times. In the first reading, focus on the situation, problems, and key players. Your goal during this reading is to operationally define the issues and problems involved in the case.

On your second reading, begin to make marginal notes reflecting your assessment of the issues presented. Differentiate important and unimportant facts, and determine where you need more information. In some cases, you will want to obtain further information (see the reading list following each case); in others, you will be able to make reasonable assumptions to fill in the gaps.

Read the case for the third time right before it is presented in class or discussed with colleagues. Your purpose at this time is to be sure that you have considered all relevant information.

Your analysis of each case should be broad. Begin with a fundamental question: What are the key issues involved in this case? Then consider the main alternatives of the case in the context of those issues and of the assigned questions. Since cases do not have a "right" answer, you should attempt to justify your decisions. In other words, your decisions must be seen to derive from your initial assumptions about key issues.

We encourage you to consider the case study questions as the *beginning* of your analysis. Use the resources suggested, as well as additional ones, to broaden your knowledge of the topics covered and thus to place the case in a wider context. And be sure to update the information provided here with further developments that have occurred since these cases were written in the fall of 1985.

CASE STUDY 1: BABY DOE

Mandating life-sustaining measures for severely disabled newborns

This case study covers an emergent health care policy concern: What is the appropriate role of the government in determining health care delivery practice? To what extent should the government be involved in clinical decision making? Should federal and state governments impose a definition of what is right for society even if it conflicts with an individual family's wishes? The far-reaching effects of these issues is demonstrated by the fact that attempts to resolve them have involved all three branches of government: executive, legislative, and judicial.

Background. Discussions of the merits of employing life-sustaining measures for severely disabled newborns are not new. Historically, these discussions took place privately between health care professionals and family members. In 1982, these private matters became a matter of public concern. In Bloomington, Indiana, the parents of an infant born with Down's syndrome and a detached esophagus made the decision, in consultation with health care professionals, to withhold from the baby life-sustaining surgical treatment. The reasons given were their reluctance to prolong the life of an infant that would no doubt meet an inevitable early death, as well as the extensive health care services that would be required to support the disabled child. Although these considerations seemed reasonable to the parents of "Baby Doe," as well as to other parents who have faced a similar decision, the Reagan Administration took exception.

Prompted by the Baby Doe case, the Department of Health and Human Services (DHHS) issued interim regulations in March 1983 regarding health care of handicapped infants. The regulations required hospitals to post in a "conspicuous place" a notice stating that, under Section 504 of the Rehabilitation Act of 1973, it is unlawful for hospitals receiving federal assistance to withhold life-sustaining treatment from a handicapped infant. They were also required to post a telephone hotline number for reporting of suspected violations of the law.

Opposition to the regulations was registered by numerous professional health care organizations, including the American Hospital Association, the American Medical Association, the ANA, the American Academy of Pediatrics, the American College of Obstetricians and Gynecologists, and the Nurses Association of the American Academy of Obstetricians and Gynecologists. This marked the first time in recent years that physicians, nurses, hospital administrators, and other health professionals have been so united in a common cause. They objected to the government's interference in clinical practice and argued that the rules did not give appropriate consideration to parents' wishes. They also pointed out that the regulations were issued with only a 15-day comment period, as opposed to the minimum of 30 days required by the Administrative Procedures Act.

In a legal challenge spearheaded by the American Academy of Pediatrics, the U.S. District Court judge for the District of Columbia described the interim rules as "arbitrary and capricious" and criticized DHHS Secretary Margaret Heckler for not appearing to give adequate consideration to the pros and cons of relying on the wishes of parents. The judge also objected to the abbreviated comment period.

After the initial set of rules was invalidated, DHHS published revised regulations and asked for public comment. The revisions still had not addressed the issues that were previously in question: government interference in clinical decision making and family wishes. At this time (November 1983), a baby was born in Stony Brook, New York, with spina bifida and hydrocephalus. In addition to the questions raised by the original Baby Doe case and the government's subsequent action, the so-called Baby Jane Doe case raised the question of whether withholding treatment to a handicapped newborn could be considered discriminatory and, furthermore, whether the government could have access to medical records in cases of possible discrimination. DHHS was denied access to this infant's records, since it was ruled and upheld that there had been no discrimination and therefore no violation.

Final regulations regarding the mandating of treatment for severely disabled newborns were issued by DHHS in January 1984. The rules included the posting of notices, the use of voluntary Infant Care Review Committees (ICRCs), and the establishment of a hotline to be used only after either the ICRC or the state child protective agency had been notified. As summarized by Secretary Heckler, the federal government was to be the "protector of last resort."

The issue has been carried over into the legislative arena as well. In 1984 Congress passed an amendment to the Child Abuse Prevention and Treatment Act that applied the definition of child abuse to cases where seriously handicapped infants were denied life-sustaining treatment. The Baby Doe provision included a detailed definition of "withholding of medically indicated treatment" that would instruct physicians, hospitals, and nurses as to when such treatment must be provided. The bill also required states that participate in the child abuse grant program to set up procedures or programs to respond to reports of medical neglect, including the withholding of medically indicated treatment. President Reagan signed the amendment on October 4, 1984.

DHHS published its final rules implementing the legislation on April 15, 1985. The final regulations were revised based on arguments from ANA and other groups that government should not further define "withholding of medically indicated treatment." Instead, HHS included the definitions as interpretive guidelines without the binding force of law. The legislation gives doctors and families the right to decide when it is appropriate to withhold care, even though the government monitors their activities.

As a result of the DHHS regulations, the states are in a position to implement their own programs, and many have done so. Louisiana was the first to sign into law the mandating of treatment for handicapped newborns.

Even though the issue has progressed in the legislative and regulatory arenas, it is still pending in the Supreme Court, which has agreed to review, during the 1985-86 term, whether Section 504 is applicable to Baby Doe cases. If the Court decides that it is, there will be two applicable pieces of legislation for cases involving disabled newborns.

Government has acted, but questions still remain. Both sides feel that they have won to a certain extent: government and right-to-life groups are pleased that action has been taken; health care professionals are pleased that they have limited the extent to which government can intervene. The issue will continue to be debated, and government, practitioners, and families are sure to be confronted with it in the future.

Case Study Questions

1. What are the health care policy problems raised by the Baby Doe case study? Outline the major positions taken by those who support the government's stand and by those who oppose it.

2. What specific protective responsibilities does society have to individuals and to society as a whole? What role does society play in curbing government's interference? What level of government (e.g., state or federal) should be responsible?

3. What interest groups were involved in the Baby Doe controversy? To what extent were they successful in achieving their ends? Why were certain groups more or less successful than others?

4. What are the "politics" of the Baby Doe case? Who stands to lose or gain in this situation? Were there any underlying reasons, ideological or political, for the government to step in?

5. What policy implications arise when the government becomes involved in social, moral, or ethical decision making?

6. What policy alternatives could the government have used other than regulation?

7. Given that the federal and state governments are mandating that care be provided to severely disabled newborns, how can this policy decision best be implemented? Who should be involved?

8. What role can nurses play in the decision-making procedures mandated by the Baby Doe regulations? What information regarding health policy and law should a nurse provide to the parents of a severely disabled newborn?

9. How much influence should interest groups have? Which groups should take precedence: those with the greatest number of adherents? those with the greatest technical expertise? those whose beliefs are in line with administrative policies?

For Further Information

ANA and AACN criticize Baby Doe regulations. (March 1985). *Capital Update, 3,* 2.

Baby Doe legislation signed by President. (October 1985). *Capital Update, 2,* 7.

Committee on the Legal and Ethical Aspects of Health Care for Children. (1983). Comments and recommendations on the "Infant Doe" proposed regulations. *Law, Medicine and Health Care, 11,* 203-209, 213.

Conferees agree on Baby Doe legislation. (September 1984). *Capital Update, 2,* 2.

Doudera, A. (1983). Section 504, handicapped newborns, and ethics committees: An alternative to the hotline. *Law, Medicine and Health Care, 11,* 200-202, 236.

Drane, J. F. (January-February 1984). The defective child: Ethical guidelines for painful dilemmas. *JOGN Nursing, 13,* 42-48.

Feldman, E., & Murray, T. H. (1984). State legislation and the handicapped newborn: A moral and political dilemma. *Law, Medicine and Health Care, 12,* 156-163.

Final Baby Doe regulations published. (April 1985). *Capital Update, 3,* 4.

Lyon, J. (1985). *Playing God in the Nursery.* New York: W. W. Norton.

New Baby Doe rule cools contoversy. (1984). *AORN Journal, 39,* 814-815.

Paris, J. J., & Fletcher, A. B. (1983). Infant Doe regulations and the absolute requirement to use nourishment and fluids for the dying infant. *Law, Medicine and Health Care, 11,* 210-213.

Solomon, S. (1984). Baby Doe cases raise questions about government role. *Nursing & Health Care, 5,* 238-239.

CASE STUDY 2

Nurse-midwives: Policy implications of the crisis in the insurance industry

This case study addresses some of the issues that can arise when a profession expands its scope of practice. This case has implications for all nurses in advanced practice but focuses on certified nurse-midwives, who for the most part have been successful in securing acceptance for their role within the health care system. However, despite their cost-effectiveness, high quality of care, and a historically low rate of liability claims, nurse-midwives have been subject to events beyond the realm of nursing practice but very much affecting their practice nonetheless.

The core of this case study is the current loss of malpractice insurance facing nurse-midwives. The situation of the nurse-midwives raises many important policy questions: To what extent should professional associations bring to the attention of government seemingly unfair practices in the private sector, especially if those practices result from forces in the economy that were not directly caused by previous government action? In other words, at what point should a problem move from the private into the public sector? As the trend continues for more nurses to practice independently, what will be the effects of the insurance crisis on other nursing specialty groups? How can they ensure that what has happened to the nurse-midwives will not happen to them, and what can they do to support the nurse-midwives?

Background. In 1955, a small group of nurse-midwives established the American College of Nurse-Midwifery (now called the American College of Nurse-Midwives, or ACNM); in 1985, there were an estimated 2,500 nurse-midwives in the United States, most of whom practice under their state's nurse practice act.

The growth in numbers of nurse-midwives and the scope of their practice is impressive. It is estimated that 3 percent of the babies in the United States are delivered by nurse-midwives, 80 percent of whom have at least a baccalaureate degree. Nurse-midwives work in clinical collaboration with physicians under written alliance and protocol agreements that establish mechanisms for consultation and referral. ACNM has an agreement with the American College of Obstetricians and Gynecologists outlining guidelines for working relationships. Approximately 75 percent of the births attended by certified nurse-midwives (CNMs) take place in hospitals; another 15 percent take place in accredited birthing centers.

The place the CNMs have created for themselves within the health care system was jeopardized when, in May 1985, ACNM was notified that its blanket malpractice insurance policy, which covered the approximately 1,400 CNMs in independent practice, would not be renewed on July 1 because of the unavailability of reinsurance. Then, in July, the insurance company further cancelled all policies that had been written after January 1, 1985. Over the next several months, ACNM contacted 17 other insurance companies but was unable to obtain insurance for its members, in spite of the nurse-midwives' low incidence of lawsuits (only 6 percent of CNMs have been sued, compared to 60 percent of obstetricians).

Indeed, this crisis for the nurse-midwives is believed to be a result not of any actions on their part but rather of a general crisis in the insurance industry that had its origin in the 1970s. During that time of high interest rates, insurance companies were eager to write policies so that they could invest the premiums at the prevailing rates of nearly 20 percent. At the same time, to attract customers, insurance premiums were kept low. In the early 1980s, this led to a crisis situation when, simultaneously, interests rates dropped sharply; insurance losses, and thus the companies' payouts, increased just as sharply; and the unrealistically low premiums failed to cover the difference. This situation is affecting several other groups, including architects, truckers, asbestos workers, towns and municipalities, and day care centers, as well as nurse-midwives, as insurance companies raise premiums and attempt to minimize risks by not writing policies.

After attempting to place their insurance with other insurance companies, ACNM pursued several other paths toward resolution of the problem. First they took the case to the states, which are responsible for regulating the insurance industry: individual nurse-midwives contacted their state insurance commissioners, legislators, and other officials. Only one state, New Jersey, was able to offer insurance through a private carrier. In other states, CNMs have obtained coverage through physician-owned companies, but these policies usually carry practice restrictions and are far more expensive than group-sponsored insurance. In New York and Texas, ACNM successfully lobbied state legislators to extend joint underwriting authority to nurse-midwives. However, the premiums for this type of insurance are prohibitively expensive (in New York, the annual premium was $72,000, whereas the average CNM's annual salary is $25,000).

In July 1985, the ANA attempted to include nurse-midwives under its personal/professional liability insurance policy for all registered nurses. Under the current plan, nurses are protected for up to $1 million per claim and $3 million each year in total claims, and the policy covers all nurses practicing within the scope of their state's nurse practice act, including nurses in expanded practice roles. The cost of this coverage is low, because the risk is spread over a large group of nurses. The ANA believed that incorporation of the nurse-midwives into a larger policy was the optimal way to resolve the crisis, because of the importance of nurse-midwifery to nursing.

The coverage was marketed to the CNM population to enthusiastic acceptance. On August 30, however, ANA was informed by their insurance broker that the insurance company would exclude nurse-midwives from the policy. ANA was able to negotiate an agreement whereby CNMs could sign up for coverage until November 1, 1985, and all existing contracts would be honored for their one-year duration.

On September 19, 1985, ACNM and ANA testified about the insurance crisis before the Subcommittee on Commerce, Transportation, and Tourism of the House Committee on Energy and Commerce. They requested that Congress authorize a federally sponsored temporary program to provide reinsurance to a private insurance company providing liability insurance for nurse-midwives. The testimony before the committee by both organizations emphasized the low rate of claims, cost-effectiveness, and benefits to medically underserved communities associated with nurse-midwifery practice.

As of November 1985, ACNM felt that it had several choices still open. Its first choice was to set up its own insurance company: in other words, for nurse-midwives to provide self-insurance for members of their profession, just as physicians do (half of malpractice policies are written by physician-owned companies). Second, the nurse-midwives might also pursue the option of attempting to secure reinsurance through the federal government for their insurance company. Third, the nurse-midwives could continue to work with the states to obtain joint underwriting authority. This process would be time-consuming because it would be necessary to go to each state individually; in addition, premiums might be high. Fourth, an attempt had been made to work through the Federal Trade Commission (FTC). The FTC works on restraint-of-trade issues. In this case they would be evaluating whether denial of insurance coverage constitutes restraint of trade.

In October 1985, the ACNM board decided to give priority to the self-insurance option. Under this plan, an ACNM insurance program would be established. Thus the problem has come full circle, and the policy issue moves, at least in part, from the public domain back into the private sector.

At the same time, however, Congress is addressing the crisis in several ways. For example, the Senate Appropriations Committee included $1 million in its fiscal year 1986 appropriations bill for the Department of Health and Human Services to investigate the issue of professional liability insurance coverage, especially for nurse-midwives. Senator Daniel Inouye (D–Hawaii) recommended language for the bill that might allow the department to begin functioning immediately as a reinsurer for nurse-midwives. Other initiatives on the insurance problem have been taken or are to be taken in the Senate Commerce Committee, the House Subcommittee on Commerce, Transportation, and Tourism (the September 19 hearings referred to above), and a presidential Insurance Task Force.

The issue is far from resolved, and it is an important one for all nurses to remain aware of and to keep their state and federal legislators informed about. There is a crisis, and the government has a role in it, even if it is only to study the matter. The current situation severely restricts the employment practice of a great many people. Even if a satisfactory solution for the nurse-midwives is reached, the situation will require ongoing monitoring and cooperation from public and private sectors to prevent a similar crisis from happening again.

Case Study Questions

1. To what do you attribute the nurse-midwives' success in gaining a place in the health-care system? Consider both clinical, social, and organizational factors.

2. Explain the causes of and reactions to the nurse-midwives' insurance problems. List recent events that have changed the situation as described in the case. Could the problems have been foreseen and forestalled?

3. Where does the responsibility for nurse-midwifery liability insurance lie? Within the government? In what branch, level, or agency? Do you agree that the government should have a role in ameliorating the crisis? Does responsibility lie in the private sector? With a professional organization or employer? Why?

4. What does this case teach other nurses with expanded practice roles? What preventive actions can they take?

5. What interest groups, both in health care and outside the health care field, would be instrumental as members of a coalition to make the nurse-midwives' request to Congress for reinsurance more effective?

6. Review the strategies the nurse-midwives have used so far. Which arguments have been effective, and with whom (government, consumers, the insurance industry)? Explain why they chose self-insurance over the other alternatives. How might they have improved their strategy?

7. Given the choice of the self-insurance route, what does a nurse-midwife in independent practice need to know before buying into the insurance policy? What information will the ACNM need to give to the public? What would a potential investor need to know about the company?

For Further Information

American College of Nurse-Midwives. (September 19, 1985). *Testimony on the scarcity and high cost of insurance.* Washington: American College of Nurse-Midwives.

American Nurses' Association. (September 19, 1985). *Testimony on the unavailability of liability insurance for nurse-midwives.* Washington: American Nurses' Association.

Bullough, B. (1985). Nurse Midwifery. *Pedicatric Nursing, 11,* 143-148.

Colburn, D. (July 3, 1985). Midwives face insurance crisis. *The Washington Post,* p. 7.

Krause, N. (1985). Supplemental report on nurse-midwifery legislation. *Journal of Nurse-Midwifery, 30,* 133-136.

Malpractice and midwives. (July 6, 1985). Editorial, *The Washington Post,* p. A18.

McCarthy, C. (July 21, 1985). Nurse-midwives and their struggle to survive. *The Washington Post,* p. B5.

Nurse-midwifery trends: Some reflections. (1985). *Journal of Nurse-Midwifery, 30,* 1-2.

Reforming malpractice law. (September 30, 1985). *Medicine & Health,* Perspectives.

Robinson, S. (1985). Role restrictions. *Nursing Times, 81,* 28-31.

Solomon, S. (1985). Diverse issues call for decisive action. *Nursing & Health Care, 6,* 479-480.

Solomon, S. (1985). D.C. regulatory battle proves our fight is far from over. *Nursing & Health Care, 6,* 242-243.

Small-Group Exercises

The purpose of these exercises is to give you a more in-depth understanding of the complexities of legislative and policy issues. They are designed for small-group discussions among three to five people but can also be done by individuals who want to understand these issues and review the exercises on their own.

The topic of the first exercise, organizing a legislative network, is critical for rallying nurses at the grassroots level. Forming a cohesive network will increase the visibility of nurses in the legislative arena. Doing this well requires careful planning and consideration of many options. The exercise is meant to point out these challenges, encourage you to evaluate your local situation, and assist you in putting together the type of network that will work best for you.

The second exercise, on the National Center for Nursing Research, is meant to increase your awareness of the questions that remain unanswered even though the legislation for the Center has been enacted. These questions relate to the processes by which the Center was established, such as the decision-making process within the nursing profession that led major nursing organizations to endorse a National Institute of Nursing and then a nursing Center. The exercise explores ways that nurses can advance nursing research on the federal level as well as the fundamental issues and definitions of nursing research, which are even more important to resolve now that the Center is a reality.

EXERCISE 1: LEGISLATIVE NETWORK

Background. You are aware of the impact that nurses have on health care legislation and policy. However, you also realize that despite the large number of nurses in your community, there is no on-going network to allow nurses to communicate effectively with legislators. A network is a formal mechanism nurses or other individuals can use to contact each other about the need to communicate with legislators at critical points in the legislative process. (For information about existing networks, contact your state nurses' association or specialty nursing organizations.)

You decide to set up a network. In order to organize properly you need to explore the following questions:

1. Who will be included in the network? Is it for nurses within your place of employment? geographic area? specialty practice? Will you include those involved in nursing education and in nursing practice?

2. Given the large number of issues that require attention, how will you determine which ones to focus on? What criteria will be used to set priorities? Will you deal with federal, state, and local issues? Which issues will have broadest appeal to the nurses in the network? Have national, state, or local nursing organizations announced positions on certain issues that may facilitate your decision making?

3. Who will be responsible for coordinating the network? one individual? a committee? If a committee, how will it be structured?

4. What structure will the network use? For example, will you use a tree-system structure or some other method of contacting participants?

5. What are realistic expectations of those participating in the network? How will people in the network be contacted if they cannot be reached by phone? How will the members of the network be kept up-to-date on issues? What will be done if someone expresses opposition to an issue being processed by the network? Who decides if and when the network should be activated?

6. How will you evaluate the effectiveness of the network?

7. What other organizations, agencies, coalitions, and so forth might you consider including as a way of branching the network and broadening the base of support?

8. One of the biggest problems in implementing a network is keeping members informed, motivated, and involved with the issues. What methods might you use to do that? Or is keeping informed the responsibility of each individual nurse? What are your strategies for expanding the network and getting other nurses involved? In other words, how will you lobby your colleagues?

EXERCISE 2: NATIONAL CENTER FOR NURSING RESEARCH

Background. In 1983, Rep. Edward Madigan (R–Illinois), ranking minority member of the House Energy and Commerce Subcommittee on Health and the Environment, proposed an amendment to legislation reauthorizing the National Institutes of Health (NIH). The bill, establishing a National Institute of Nursing at NIH, challenged many of nursing's most ardent legislative supporters, such as Rep. Henry Waxman (D–California), chairman of the subcommittee, by forcing them to come to terms with both their previous commitments to oppose any new institutes at NIH and their longstanding legislative support of nursing. Ultimately, with Rep. Waxman's critical support, the bill passed the House unanimously in November 1983.

On the Senate side, Senator Orrin Hatch (R–Utah), chairman of the Senate Labor and Human Resources Committee, initially wavered but eventually supported the House version of the nursing institute bill. Despite approval by both houses of Congress, President Reagan vetoed the entire NIH bill in October 1984.

In 1985, Rep. Madigan, with the consensus of the major nursing organizations that supported the bill, agreed to yield to the Administration's objections to an institute and proposed instead the establishment of a National Center for Nursing Research at NIH. Despite Congressional approval of the bill, President Reagan vetoed the entire NIH bill once again. But this time, Congress overrode the veto, making the National Center for Nursing Research a reality.

Issues. The process of establishing a new nursing research structure, whether institute or center, at NIH is the result of a variety of factors, both external and internal to the nursing community. In addition, the process through which the Nursing Tri-Council (ANA, NLN, and AACN) decided to endorse the Institute raised questions about the methods that nursing associations use to decide upon endorsement of a particular issue. Given this background, here are some questions for discussion:

1. What is the definition of nursing research? Is it to be done by nurses only? If not, who else is qualified to conduct nursing research? What implications does this have for establishing a nursing research center at NIH? (In other words, how should the parameters of nursing research be determined?) How important is this issue to the future of nursing?

2. How does nursing research fit into the purpose and mission of NIH?

3. In the future, how might associations in the Nursing Tri-Council decide whether or not to endorse a proposal such as the National Institute of Nursing, especially in view of the short amount of time they have to make such decisions? How are they then accountable to their members? What about the members' obligations to delegate such decisions to their elected or appointed officers? What is the appropriate balance of power?

4. What were the pros and cons of placing a national center for nursing research within NIH?

5. In view of the need to give nursing research more visibility within the federal government, what other alternatives, besides a nursing institute, were considered? What are the advantages and disadvantages of the alternatives? Or, what other information do you need before responding to this question?

6. What should nurses, especially nurse researchers, do to advance nursing research at the federal level? Include in your answer activities within and beyond NIH.

7. What kinds of data and information on nursing and nursing research are needed to strengthen our efforts to promote nursing research at the federal level?

8. What is your action plan for educating your colleagues and becoming more involved in discussions pertaining to nursing research?

9. Now that the Center has been approved, what challenges will nurses face in setting it up and implementing a nursing research program at NIH?

Resource List

The following lists are representative samplings of resources available in the following categories: books, newspapers, newsletters, periodicals, government sources, audiovisual materials, and experiences (primarily internships). Addresses and telephone numbers are provided for all sources given, except book publishers.

As a student of policy, you should be familiar with three general types of resources. The first is books that provide background information on such topics as politics, political and economic theory, and policy analysis. Many text books fall into this category, but other books of interest are listed here as well.

Second, you should become familiar with a wide variety of periodical literature, such as newspapers, journals, and newsletters. It is important for policy students to read a national newspaper, such as the *New York Times* or *Washington Post*, regularly. Equally important, you should begin to absorb the range of opinion represented in the policy journals, both in nursing and other fields, and the variety of viewpoints presented in special-interest newsletters. These resources are a supplement to, rather than a substitute for, the basic information gathered from books.

The third type of resource is direct experience, either the formal sort obtained through a fellowship or internship or the informal experience obtained through actual participation in the policy proces. Nursing organizations provide the most likely opportunity for students to get involved, in such ways as lobbying, presenting testimony, writing and telephoning legislators, petitioning, and so forth. Needless to say, you should have a thorough background in the political process and an understanding of policy making before you attempt direct action.

The resources provided here, especially journals and newsletters, are a representative sample, not an exhaustive list. You will probably find many others in your own library, and you should examine as many as possible at least once and begin to read several on a regular basis. Many of the private organizations listed here publish newsletters and other policy-related documents. From government sources, notably the Government Printing Office, you can obtain copies of the *Federal Register* and *Congressional Register*, as well as many other documents.

A brief list of sources for audiovisual materials on policy and politics is provided, as well as a more extensive list of organizations that sponsor policy internships and fellowships open to nurses. Write to these agencies for specific information about the experiences and eligibility requirements.

BOOKS

Following are three lists of books. "Best sellers" are the ten books most often used as texts in policy couses. "Classics" are the standard reference works in the field. Every student of policy should, ideally, be familiar with these works. Finally, the "Background Reading" list contains basic references that will provide information to both student and instructor.

Best Sellers

Aiken, L. H. (Ed). (1981). *Health Policy and Nursing Practice*. New York: McGraw-Hill.

Aiken, L., & Gortner, S. (Eds). (1982). *Nursing in the 1980s: Crises, Opportunities, Challenges*. Philadelphia: J. B. Lippincott.

American Nurses' Association. (1980). *Nursing: A Social Policy Statement*. Kansas City: American Nurses' Association.

Feldstein, P. (1979). *Health Care Economics*. New York: John Wiley & Sons.

Fuchs, V. (1982). *Who Shall Live? Health, Economics and Social Choices*. New York: Basic Books.

Kalisch, B. J., & Kalisch, P. A. (1982). *Politics of Nursing*. Philadelphia: J. B. Lippincott.

Litman, T. J., & Robbins, L. S. (Eds). (1984). *Health Politics and Policy*. New York: John Wiley & Sons.

Milio, N. (1981). *Promoting Health through Public Policy*. Philadelphia: F. A. Davis.

Redman, E. (1978). *The Dance of Legislation*. New York: Simon and Schuster.

Starr, P. (1982). *The Social Transformation of American Medicine*. New York: Basic Books.

Classics

Aaron, H., & Schwartz, W. (1984). *Painful Prescription: Rationing Hospital Care*. Washington, D.C.: Brookings Institution.

Ashley, J. A. (1976). *Hospitals, Paternalism, and the Role of the Nurse*. New York: Teachers College Press.

Davis, K., & Schoen, C. (1978). *Health and the War on Poverty: A Ten Year Appraisal*. Washington, D.C.: Brookings Institution.

Dahl, R. (1976). *Modern Political Analysis*. Englewood Cliffs, N. J: Prentice-Hall.

Dror, Y. (1971). *Design for Policy Sciences*. New York: Elsevier.

Ehrenreich, B., & English, D. (1973). *Witches, Midwives and Nurses: A History of Women Healers*. Westbury, New York: The Feminist Press.

Institute of Medicine. (1983). *Nursing and Nursing Education: Public Policies and Private Actions*. Washington, D.C.: National Academy Press.

Kalisch, B. J., & Kalisch, P. A. (1978). *The Advance of American Nursing*. Boston: Little, Brown.

Knowles, J. (Ed). (1977). *Doing Better, Feeling Worse: Health in the United States*. New York: Norton.

Lasswell, R. (1958). *Politics: Who Gets What, When, How.* New York: Peter Smith.

Lindblom, C. E. (1968). *The Policymaking Process.* Englewood Cliffs, N.J.: Prentice-Hall.

Nakamura, R., & Smallwood, F. (1980). *The Politics of Policy Implementation.* New York: St. Martin's.

Navarro, V. (Ed). (1981). *Imperialism, Health and Medicine.* Farmingdale, NY: Baywood Publishing Company.

Thompson, F. (1983). *Health Policy and the Bureaucracy.* Cambridge, MA: MIT Press.

Verba, F., & Nie, N. H. (1972). *Participation in America: Political Democracy and Social Equality.* New York: Harper & Row.

Wildavsky, A. (1979). *The Politics of the Budgetary Process.* Boston: Little, Brown.

Wildavsky, A. (1979). *Speaking Truth to Power: The Art and Craft of Policy Analysis.* Boston: Little, Brown.

Background Reading

Bagwell, M., & Clements, S. (1985). *A Political Handbook for Health Professionals.* Boston: Little, Brown.

Blau, P. M. (1967). *Exchange and Power in Social Life.* New York: John Wiley & Sons

Christenson, R. M., Engel, A. S., Jacobs, D. N., Rejai, M., & Waltzer, H. (1972). *Ideologies and Modern Politics.* New York: Dodd, Mead.

Dye, T. R. (1976). *Policy Analysis.* Birmingham: University of Alabama Press.

Enthoven, A. (1980). *Health Plan.* Reading, MA: Addison-Wesley.

Friedson, E. (1970). *Professional Dominance: The Social Structure of Medical Care.* New York: Atherton Press.

Grissum, M., & Spengler, C. (1976). *Womanpower and Health Care.* Boston: Little, Brown.

Lindblom, C. E. (1977). *Politics and Markets.* New York: Basic Books.

Lee, P. R., Estes, C. L., & Ramsay, N. B. (Eds). (1984). *The Nation's Health.* San Francisco: Boyd & Fraser.

Marmor, T. (1973). *The Politics of Medicare.* Chicago: Aldine Publishing Company.

Marmor, T. R., & Christianson, J. B. (1982). *Health Care Policy: A Political Economy Approach.* Beverly Hills: Sage Publications.

Mason, D., & Talbott, S. (1985). *Political Action Handbook for Nurses.* Menlo Park, CA: Addison-Wesley.

Mechanic, D. (1983). *Handbook of Health, Health Care and the Health Professions.* New York: The Free Press.

Mezey, M., & McGivern, D. (Eds). (1985). *Nurses, Nurse Practitioners.* Boston: Little, Brown.

Quade, E. S. (1982). *Analysis for Public Decisions.* New York: Elsevier.

Samuelson, P. (1985). *Economics,* 12th ed. New York: McGraw-Hill.

Shaw, L. E. (Ed). (1973). *Modern Competing Ideologies.* Lexington, KY: D. C. Heath.

Somers, A. R. (1971). *Health Care in Transition: Directions for the Future.* Chicago: Hospital Research and Educational Trust.

Somers, A. R., & Somers, H. M. (1977). *Health and Health Care Policies in Perspective.* Germantown, MD: Aspen.

Vane, C. (1975). *A Guide to Library Sources in Political Science: American Government.* Washington, D.C.: American Political Science Association.

NEWSPAPERS

The New York Times
229 West 43rd Street
New York, New York 10036

The Wall Street Journal
200 Burnett Road
Chicopee, Massachusetts 01021
(413) 592-7761

The Washington Post
Mail Subscription Department
1150 15th Street, N.W.
Washington, D.C. 20071
(800) 424-9203

Washington Post National Weekly Edition
1150 15th Street, N.W.
Washington, D.C. 20071
(800) 624-2367 ext. 4280

NEWSLETTERS

Washington Report on Medicine & Health
and
Washington Report on Health Legislation
McGraw-Hill Book Company
1120 Vermont Avenue, N.W.
Suite 1200
Washington, D.C. 20005

Legislative Updates and other periodic
publications
National League for Nursing
10 Columbus Circle
New York, N.Y. 10019-1350

Capital Update
ANA Washington Office
1101 14th Street, N.W.
Washington, D.C. 20005

The Political Nurse
ANA Department of Political Education
1101 14th Street, N.W.
Washington, D.C. 20005

Legislative Network for Nurses
Legislative Network for Nursing, Inc.
P.O. Box 44071
L'Enfant Plaza, S.W.
Washington, D.C. 20026

PRIVATE ORGANIZATIONS AND GOVERNMENT SOURCES

American Association of Retired Persons
1909 K Street, N.W.
Washington, D.C. 20049
(202) 872-4700

American Hospital Association
444 North Capitol Street, N.W.
Suite 550
Washington, D.C. 20001
(202) 638-1100

American Medical Association
1101 Vermont Avenue, N.W.
Washington, D.C. 20005
(202) 789-7400

American Medical Peer Review Association
440 First Street, N.W.
Suite 500
Washington, D.C. 20001
(202) 628-1853

American Political Science Association
1527 New Hampshire Avenue, N.W.
Washington, D.C. 20036
(202) 483-2512

American Psychological Association
1200 17th Street, N.W.
Washington, D.C. 20036
(202) 955-7660

American Public Health Association
1015 15th Street, N.W.
Washington, D.C. 20005
(202) 789-5600

Children's Defense Fund
122 C Street, N.W.
Suite 400
Washington, D.C. 20001
(202) 628-8787

Congressional Budget Office
HOB Annex #2
Washington, D.C. 20515
(202) 226-2600

*Congressional Record, Federal Register,
Digest of Public General Bills and
Resolutions*
Superintendent of Documents
Government Printing Office
Washington, D.C. 20402
(202) 783-3238

Congressional Research Service
101 Independence Avenue, S.E.
Washington, D.C. 20540
(202) 287-5700

General Accounting Office
Headquarters:
441 G Street, N.W.
Washington, D.C. 20548
(202) 275-2812 (Office of Public Information/Press)
Ordering reports:
P.O. Box 6015
Gaithersburg, MD 20877
(202) 275-6241

Government Printing Office
Superintendent of Documents
710 North Capitol Street, N.W.
Washington, D.C. 20402
(202) 275-3204 (information)
(202) 783-3238 (publications orders and inquiries)

House Document Room
H226, Capitol
Washington, D.C. 20515
(202) 225-3456

Institute of Medicine
2101 Constitution Avenue, N.W.
Washington, D.C. 20418
(202) 334-2169

National Health Council, Inc.
622 Third Avenue
New York, New York 10017
(212) 972-2700

Office of Technology Assessment
U.S. Congress
Washington, D.C. 20540
(202) 287-5580

Prospective Payment Assessment Commission
300 Seventh Street, S.W.
Washington, D.C. 20024
(202) 453-3986

Senate Document Room
SH-B04
Senate Hart Office Building
Washington, D.C. 20510
(202) 224-7860

PERIODICALS

American Journal of Public Health
American Public Health Association
1015 15th Street, N.W.
Washington, D.C. 20005
(202) 789-5600

The American Political Science Review
American Political Science Association
1527 New Hampshire Avenue, N.W.
Washington, D.C. 20036
(202) 483-2512

Congressional Quarterly Service and
Guide to Congress
Weekly Report
Congressional Quarterly, Inc.
1414 22nd Street, N.W.
Washington, D.C. 20037

Economics and Business Letter
Slippery Rock State College
Department of Economics and Business
Slippery Rock, PA 16057

Health Affairs
Project HOPE
Millwood, VA 22646
(703) 837-2100

Health Care Financing Review
Health Care Financing Administration
Department of Health & Human Services
East High Rise Building, Room 365
6401 Security Blvd.
Baltimore, MD 21207
(301) 597-3000
Subscribe to:
Superintendent of Documents
Washington, D.C. 20402

Inquiry
Blue Cross & Blue Shield Association
676 North St. Clair Street
Chicago, IL 60611
Subscribe to:
Box 527
Glenview, IL 60025

J.E.I. (Journal of Economic Issues)
Association for Evolutionary Economics
c/o F. Gregory Hayden
Department of Economics
University of Nebraska
Lincoln, Nebraska 68588
(202) 822-7845

Journal of Health Politics, Policy and Law
    Duke University
    Department of Health Administration
    Box 3018
    Durham, NC 27710
    (919) 684-4188

Journal of Policy Analysis and
Management
    Association for Public Policy Analysis
    and Management
    John Wiley & Sons, Inc.
    605 Third Avenue
    New York, NY 10016
    (202) 692-6000

Journal of Public Health Policy
    Journal of Public Health Policy, Inc.
    23 Pheasant Way
    South Burlington, VT 05401

Milbank Memorial Fund Quarterly
    Cambridge University Press
    510 North Avenue
    New Rochelle, NY 10801
    (914) 235-0300

Modern Healthcare
    Crain Communications
    740 Rush Street
    Chicago, IL 60611

National Journal
    Government Research Corporation
    1730 M Street, N.W.
    Washington, D.C. 20036
    (202) 857-1400

Nursing Economics
    Anthony J. Jannetti, Inc.
    North Woodbury Road
    Box 56
    Pitman, NJ 08071
    (609) 589-2319

Nursing & Health Care
    National League for Nursing
    10 Columbus Circle
    New York, NY 10019-1350
    (212) 582-1022

Nursing Outlook
    American Journal of Nursing Company
    555 West 57th Street
    New York, NY 10019
    (212) 582-8820

Policy Sciences
    Elsevier Scientific Publications Company
    Box 211
    1000 AE Amsterdam
    Netherlands

Policy Studies Review
    Policy Studies Organization
    University of Illinois
    361 Lincoln Hall
    Urbana, IL 61801
    (217) 359-8541

Public Administration Review
    American Society for Public
    Administration
    1120 G Street, N.W.
    Suite 500
    Washington, D.C. 20005
    (202) 393-7878

Public Choice
    Kluwer Academic Publishers Group
    Distribution Center
    Box 322
    3300 AH Dordrecht
    Netherlands

Social Policy
    Social Policy Corporation
    33 West 42nd Street
    New York, NY 10036
    (212) 840-7619

AUDIOVISUAL MATERIALS

DRGs: A New Era for Nursing (videotape)
    National League for Nursing
    10 Columbus Circle
    New York, NY 10019-1350

Nurses, Politics, and Public Policy
(videotape)
    American Nurses' Association
    2420 Pershing Road
    Kansas City, MO 64108
    (816) 474-5720
    (also available from the state nurses'
    association)

League of Women Voters of the United
States
    1730 M Street, N.W.
    Washington, D.C. 20036
    (202) 429-1965

National Women's Educational Fund
1410 Q Street, N.W.
Washington, D.C. 20009
(202) 462-8606

EXPERIENCES

American Association for the Advancement of Science
AAAS Congressional Science &
Engineering Fellows Program
1515 Massachusetts Avenue, N.W.
Washington, D.C. 20005
(202) 467-4400

American Association of Colleges of Nursing
One Dupont Circle
Suite 530
Washington, D.C. 20036
(202) 463-6930

American Association of Retired Persons
1909 K Street, N.W.
Washington, D.C. 20049
(202) 872-4700

American Hospital Association
444 N. Capitol Street, N.W.
Suite 550
Washington, D.C. 20001
(202) 638-1100

American Nurses' Association
Washington Office
1101 14th Street, N.W.
Suite 200
Washington, D.C. 20005
(202) 789-1800

American Political Science Association
1527 New Hampshire Avenue, N.W.
Washington, D.C. 20036
(202) 483-2512

American Society for Nursing Service Administration
840 North Lakeshore Drive
Chicago, IL 60611
(312) 280-6410

National Advisory Council on Women's Educational Programs
425 13th Street, N.W.
Washington, D.C. 20004
(202) 376-1038

National Governors Association
444 North Capitol Street
Suite 250
Washington, D.C. 20001
(202) 624-5300

National Hospice Organization
1901 North Fort Meyer Drive
Suite 402
Arlington, VA 22209
(202) 243-5900

Robert Wood Johnson Health Policy Fellowship Program
Institute of Medicine
2101 Constitution Avenue
Washington, D.C. 20418
(202) 389-6891

White House Fellowship Program
712 Jackson Place, N.W.
Washington, D.C. 20503
(202) 395-4522

Women's Research and Education Institute
204 Fourth Street, S.E.
Washington, D.C. 20003
(202) 546-1090

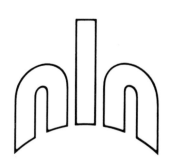

National League for Nursing
10 Columbus Circle
New York, New York 10019-1350

Pub. No. 15-1995A   7.5M-0186-07950   ISBN 0-88737-224-4